Cognitive–Behavioural Interventions in

Physiotherapy and Occupational Therapy

D1581556

For Elsevier:

Publisher: **Heidi Harrison**

Associate Editor: **Siobhan Campbell**

Project Manager: **Christine Johnston**

Design: **Charles Gray**

Illustration Manager: **Gillian Richards**

Illustrator: **David Gardner**

Cognitive–Behavioural Interventions in
Physiotherapy and Occupational Therapy

Edited by

Marie Donaghy PhD BA(Hons) FCSP ILTM FHEA
Professor of Physiotherapy,
Dean of School of Health Sciences
Queen Margaret University, Edinburgh, UK

Maggie Nicol PhD MPhil FCOT Cert FE Dip COT
Professor of Occupational Therapy,
Head of Occupational Therapy
Queen Margaret University, Edinburgh, UK

Kate Davidson PhD CPsychol FBPsS
Professor of Psychology,
Director of Glasgow Institute of Psychosocial
Interventions, University of Glasgow,
Gartnavel Royal Hospital, Glasgow, UK

Foreword by

Paul M Salkovskis BSc MPhil (Clin Psychol)
PhD C Psychol FBPsS
Professor of Clinical Psychology and Applied Science,
Institute of Psychiatry, King's College, London, UK
Clinical Director, Maudsley Hospital Centre for
Anxiety Disorders and Trauma, South London and
Maudsley Foundation Trust, London, UK

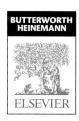

EDINBURGH LONDON NEW YORK OXFORD PHILADELPHIA ST LOUIS SYDNEY TORONTO 2008

BUTTERWORTH
HEINEMANN
ELSEVIER

An imprint of Elsevier Limited

First published 2008

© 2008, Elsevier Ltd

ISBN-13: 9780750688000

British Library Cataloguing in Publication Data
A catalogue record for this book is available from the British Library.

Library of Congress Cataloging in Publication Data
A catalog record for this book is available from the Library of Congress.

Note
Neither the Publisher nor the Authors assume any responsibility for any loss or injury and/or damage to persons or property arising out of or related to any use of the material contained in this book. It is the responsibility of the treating practitioner, relying on independent expertise and knowledge of the patient, to determine the best treatment and method of application for the patient.

The Publisher

 ELSEVIER your source for books, journals and multimedia in the health sciences
www.elsevierhealth.com

Working together to grow
libraries in developing countries

www.elsevier.com | www.bookaid.org | www.sabre.org

ELSEVIER   BOOK AID International   Sabre Foundation

Printed in China

The publisher's policy is to use paper manufactured from sustainable forests

Contents

v

Contributors

Kate Davidson PhD CPsychol FBPsS
Professor of Psychology, Director of Glasgow Institute of Psychosocial Interventions,
University of Glasgow, Gartnavel Royal Hospital, Glasgow, UK

Marie Donaghy PhD BA(Hons) FCSP ILTM FHEA
Professor of Physiotherapy, Dean of School of Health Sciences, Queen Margaret University,
Edinburgh, UK

Edward A S Duncan PhD BSc(Hons) Dip CBT
Clinical Research Fellow Nursing Midwifery and Allied Health Professions Research Unit,
University of Stirling, Stirling, UK

Tina Everett MSc MCSP
Specialist Physiotherapist, Oxford, UK

Jan S Gill PhD BSc(Hons) ILTM
Senior Lecturer in Physiology and Pharmacology, School of Health Sciences,
Queen Margaret University, Edinburgh, UK

Anne Joice Dip COT MSc
Head Occupational Therapist, Cognitive Behavioural Therapist, STEPS Primary Care Mental
Health Team, Glasgow, UK

Liz Macleod BSc(Hons) MCSP
Pain Management Specialist, Forth Valley Health Board, UK

Denis Martin DPhil MSc BSc(Hons) MCSP
Reader in Rehabilitation School of Health and Social Care, University of Teesside,
Middlesbrough, UK

Maggie Nicol PhD MPhil FCOT Cert FE Dip COT
Professor in Occupational Therapy, Head of Occupational Therapy, Queen Margaret
University, Edinburgh, UK

George E Ralston PhD MAppSci BA(Hons) PgDipBus AFBPsS MiMgt
Area Consultant Clinical Psychologist, Glasgow, UK

Mick Skelly MSc MCSP Dip Phys Dip AD
Superintendent Physiotherapist, Rosslynlee Hospital, Roslin, Midlothian, UK

Anne Stewart MB BS BSc MRCPsych
Consultant Adolescent Psychiatrist, Oxford City Child and Adolescent Mental Health
Service, Park Hospital, Oxford, UK
Senior Clinical Lecturer, University of Oxford, Oxford, UK

Foreword

Cognitive–Behavioural Therapy is Evidence Based . . . and more.

Cognitive–behavioural therapy (CBT) works, it works well, it works comprehensively and its effectiveness has been clearly demonstrated. This is not true for any other psychological approach to therapy, yet most psychological therapy is not CBT, and most professionals are not being trained in CBT. Why, in the era of 'evidence based approaches', is this still so? At its simplest, there is a problem of dissemination, an important problem for which this book is an important part of the solution.

There are, of course, other factors. CBT is still relatively new, and despite overwhelming evidence of both efficacy and effectiveness, clinical inertia and conservatism has been and still is very strong. Professionals often forget just how new this approach is, not least because of the huge scientific impact it has made. It is no exaggeration to say that, were it not for behavioural and cognitive–behavioural therapies, psychological therapy would be regarded as, at best, largely ineffective (see Roth & Fonagy 1996), and at worst a potentially harmful waste of patient time and professional resources.

It is symptomatic of the problem that, although research evidence for both the effectiveness and theoretical underpinnings of behaviour therapy and then cognitive–behavioural therapy began to appear in the 1960s and 70s, translation into practice in any significant way has taken much longer. Early work was mostly confined to problems where overt behaviour could be targeted (see Chapter 1). CBT has only really become a serious contender in terms of health service based delivery of psychological therapy over the past twenty years with the theoretical and practical integration of cognitive and behavioural strategies (Salkovskis 1996). The first applications of *cognitive* approaches focused on 'the common cold of Psychiatry', depression (Beck 1979), with this still being a key area (see Chapter 4). Research subsequently led to the expansion of this approach into aspects of anxiety where changing behaviour (as in exposure and operant approaches) was less likely to be effective, requiring the understanding and modification of the negative thinking which drove mood changes and motivated problematic behaviours (Clark 1999). Over the same period, work conducted on an ever wider range of clinical conditions indicated the importance of specificity in the understanding and efficient treatment not only of psychological problems but also psychological aspects of physical problems, some of which are described in part two of this book. Cognitive–behaviour therapy has evolved into cognitive–behavioural therapies, with the treatment of depression being carried out quite differently from the treatment of bulimia nervosa, obsessive compulsive disorder and so on.

The pace of change has brought problems as well as promise. Competent CBT practitioners were thin on the ground, and jealous detractors and opponents have been common and vocal. By the first decade of this century, the imbalance of empirical support for CBT, by contrast with most other forms of psychotherapy, had become so embarrassing that it became impossible to ignore. Bizarrely, some have sought to completely reject the notion of evidence in psychological treatment, claiming that the whole idea is mistaken (Marzillier 2004). It has been suggested that CBT is 'mechanistic', dealing with symptoms rather than 'the whole person'. Such critics seem to equate the use of empirically grounded strategies to help people change as somehow resulting in a detached position. As readers of this book will know, the exact opposite is true; that is, good therapy involves taking the empirically grounded expertise of the therapist and flexibly merging it with the patient's understanding of their situation and problem. This process leads to the collaborative development of a formulation, where patient and therapist work together to reach a shared understanding of the person's problems and how they can best be managed, as clearly described throughout this book. The failure to balance evidence on the one hand with the patient's values and experience on the other at best represents bad practice, and at worst might be regarded as professional negligence.

Other critics claim that CBT is appropriate for 'simple' cases, but that more complex problems require a different, more complex approach. Quite apart from the fact that there is now extremely good evidence that CBT is highly effective for a range of complex problems (readily illustrated by the many examples given in this book), there is an obvious flaw in this premise. Given that psychological treatments 'of a more complex nature' have not been found to be effective for simple problems, how can we then assume that they will be effective for more complex cases? The reality is that CBT has progressed by reducing apparently complex problems to their (often) simpler elements, with treatment being carried out on the basis of evolving formulations. Such formulations are modified according to individual patient responses guided by empirically validated concepts rather than being dogmatically tied to them. This process, helping the patients to make sense of their problems in ways which allow them to choose to change rather than being overwhelmed by the confusing nature of their problems, is itself a complex skill, and complexity should be neither ignored nor exaggerated. Therapy should be as simple as possible and no simpler.

What, then, is the 'secret' of the success of CBT? It is my view that the key to understanding the basis of current CBT applications lies in two areas. Firstly, CBT emphasises the importance of helping the patient to deal with factors involved in the *maintenance* of their clinical problems. For example, everyone becomes sad from time to time, especially when bad things happen; however, clinical depression involves more prolonged episodes, in which particular patterns of distorted (negative) thinking and resulting problematic and counter-productive behaviours have prevented the normal process of recovery. Similar maintaining factors have been identified by systematic research into a wide range of specific problems. Experimental and clinical research on both specific and general maintaining factors has been used to evaluate the most important targets for CBT treatment and how these can be modified.

Secondly, identifying specificity across different clinical problems has been crucial. Although the cognitive–behavioural theories and therapies used today have important trans-diagnostic elements, research findings also make it clear that there are important differences between clinical problems which require that specific strategies be flexibly applied. It is this flexible and person-centred application of theoretical and empirical work which has proven effective, efficient and empowering

x

for the people we seek to help. CBT is more than evidence based; it is an empirically grounded clinical intervention (Salkovskis 2002).

However, the expansion of CBT into new areas and the application of a wide range of different clinical problems also presents a new set of problems. Demand for CBT has massively outstripped the supply of adequately trained practitioners. To add to this problem, CBT is rapidly evolving, requiring practitioners to constantly update and hone their skills. No therapist can acquire the full range of CBT skills required for the treatment of the full range of anxiety disorders, depression, pain syndromes, enduring mental illness, eating disorders, substance misuse and so on (and on . . .). However, solutions are at hand in terms of concepts of stepped care and specific training (see Chapter 11). Last, but not least, solutions will increasingly be found in therapists developing expertise in empowering service users to more effectively apply CBT. As patients appropriately seek to take control of key health issues, CBT will become a key part of Evidence Based Patient Choice. This book should help those who read it gain the understanding that they need not only to help patients who come to them in need but also to empower them to make best use of such help. CBT is ultimately about helping people to find more effective ways of helping themselves, a concept entirely familiar to the readers of this book.

Paul M Salkovskis

References

Beck A T 1979 Cognitive therapy of depression. Guilford Press, New York

Clark D M 1999 Anxiety disorders: Why they persist and how to treat them. Behaviour Research and Therapy 37(S1):S5–S28

Marzillier J 2004 The myth of evidence-based psychotherapy. The Psychologist 17:392–395

Roth A, Fonagy P 1996 What works for whom? Guilford Press, New York

Salkovskis P M 1996 Resolving the cognition-behaviour debate. In Salkovskis P M (ed) Trends in cognitive-behaviour therapy. John Wiley, Chichester

Salkovskis P M 2002 Empirically grounded clinical interventions: Cognitive–behavioural therapy progesses through a multi-dimensional approach to clinical science. Behavioural and Cognitive Psychotherapy 30:3–9

Introduction

What is the purpose of this book?

The purpose of the book is to increase knowledge and awareness of how cognitive–behavioural interventions can be applied within a theoretical framework from which physiotherapists and occupational therapists work. The book explains the psychological model and provides a rationale for applying cognitive–behavioural therapy (CBT) as a tool to strengthen physiotherapy and occupational therapy interventions.

Who will use this book?

This book is designed primarily for students and practitioners of occupational therapy and physiotherapy but will also be useful for nurses and other health-care professions who apply cognitive–behavioural interventions in their work.

This is not just another cognitive–behavioural therapy book. The book is about the profession of physiotherapy and occupational therapy stating the parameters for application of cognitive–behavioural interventions and explaining how this links with models of practice of occupational therapy and physiotherapy.

The book is not designed to create experts in cognitive–behavioural therapy but to enhance the ability of occupational therapists and physiotherapists to more effectively apply appropriate cognitive–behavioural interventions with individuals who experience a wide variety of disorders.

Why do occupational therapists and physiotherapists need to be knowledgeable about cognitive–behavioural interventions?

Psychological models form an increasingly important part of the theoretical knowledge base applied to practice in occupational therapy and physiotherapy and this is highlighted at national conferences and in recent research publications. However, the articulation of how psychological models are applied in occupational therapy and physiotherapy has not been debated in the professional literature. With an increasing emphasis on evidence-based practice both physiotherapy and occupational therapy recognize the need to utilize interventions originally derived from other disciplines such as cognitive–behavioural therapy, which has an evidence base extending back twenty years, particularly in mental health.

The difference between cognitive–behavioural therapy as a treatment intervention in its own right and the use of cognitive–behavioural strategies to enhance another therapeutic intervention needs to be clearly distinguished.

In what areas of occupational therapy and physiotherapy are cognitive–behavioural interventions helpful?

Occupational therapists and physiotherapists are using cognitive–behavioural therapy in two main areas.

1. In mental health, cognitive–behavioural interventions in affective disorders and anxiety, addictions and, to a lesser extent, in enduring mental illness have been found to be helpful.
2. Chronic pain: fibromyalgia and chronic fatigue. Chronic pain in particular has been an important area of development for both occupational therapists and physiotherapists.

What will I learn by reading this book?

The book is in two parts.

Part One opens with an introduction to cognitive–behavioural therapy allowing the reader to become familiar with key concepts. There follows the application of the cognitive–behavioural interventions within occupational therapy and physiotherapy where models of practice are explored within the discipline specific and interdisciplinary context. Case studies are used to illustrate these models. The biomedical links between cognitions and behaviour are explored in recognition that mental processes are only made possible by the 'hardware' of the nervous system. The importance of this section is to facilitate a wider understanding of the complexities of the interaction between the brain, the body, beliefs, emotions and behaviour.

Part Two is more practical. It focuses on how cognitive–behavioural interventions are applied to specific problems or disorders. The evidence base for the application of cognitive–behavioural interventions is referred to in each chapter. The evidence base is better developed in some areas compared to others.

In each of these more applied chapters, we have tried to illustrate the application of interventions by case studies or case vignettes. These examples have been created from clinical experience rather than being identified with one particular person. The names used in the case studies bear no relation to any particular individual.

The contributing authors come from a variety of disciplines. This, in some way, illustrates the broad applicability of cognitive–behavioural interventions. We believe that anyone who works in a health context can benefit from reading this book, as it will develop ideas and understanding of how to apply cognitive–behavioural interventions.

Part Two starts with a focus on mental health and opens with a chapter on cognitive–behavioural therapy for depression which includes a fuller case study to give the reader a more detailed account of the application of cognitive therapy. We strongly recommend that this chapter is read first as it provides a thorough and clear account of how CBT can be applied with an individual and will aid readers unfamiliar with this model to a deeper understanding of the CBT process. The focus shifts to provide application to a selection of other commonly encountered disorders. All of the remaining chapters have case vignettes which, although briefer, nonetheless highlight the specific focus of the clinical syndrome and application without being repetitive. We recognize that the clinical areas covered in this section do not constitute an exhaustive list of CBT applications for occupational therapists and physiotherapists but allow the reader to gain an understanding of how CBT can be applied to individuals with a wide variety of disorders.

Marie, Maggie and Kate

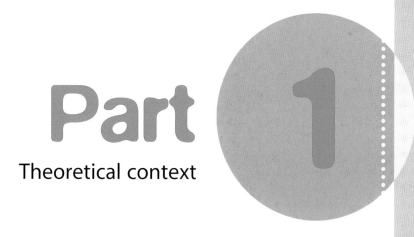

Part

Theoretical context

Cognitive–behavioural therapy: origins and developments

Kate Davidson

The origins of cognitive–behavioural therapy

A T Beck, the founder of cognitive–behavioural therapy, was born in 1921 in the United States. He was educated in New England and studied at Brown University before graduating from Yale School of Medicine (Weishaar 1993). Beck completed his analytic training in 1958 at the time when psychoanalytic therapy was the dominant model of psychotherapy in the United States. Beck's observations of a patient's thoughts and feelings did not seem to fit with psychoanalytic theory. He found evidence from studying the dreams of depressed and non-depressed patients, and from interviews with depressed patients, that depressed patients made specific errors in the content and form of thinking that indicated a general negative bias towards self, others and the world (Beck & Ward 1961, Beck 1963). In addition, he observed that patients described themes concerning being defeated and overwhelmed rather than, as psychoanalytic theory would have predicted, sadomasochistic themes. In psychoanalytic theory, depression was thought to be caused by self-directed hostility or anger turned in onto the self. Beck concluded that depression was characterized by a consistent negative bias towards the self, the world and the future. From these early findings, he developed a more general theory of the emotional disorders in which the appraisal of information about the environment was central.

Against this backdrop, other psychological theories and therapies were being developed that were also to change the way in which human problems were construed in the latter half of the twentieth century. In particular, behaviour therapy, with its roots in learning theories, was proving useful in treating neurotic disorders. Hans Eysenck, an early developer of behaviour therapy in the UK, challenged the evidence for the efficacy of psychoanalytic therapy. He argued that neuroses were not caused by unconscious conflicts and that symptoms or disturbed behaviours were the 'real' problem rather than a manifestation of an underlying problem. Behaviours were regarded as being learned and therefore could be unlearned. Unlike psychoanalytic thinkers, behaviour theorists thought that if symptoms could be got rid of, then the person was 'cured' and no longer suffering from neurosis.

In parallel, in the United States a number of psychologists were developing Skinner's ideas on operant conditioning to clinical problems. An individual's behaviour could be changed by systematically rewarding a specific response or by withholding a reward if it was not the desired response. Based on these findings, token economies were introduced to hospital wards of chronically institutionalized individuals with severe mental health problems. Patient behaviours were systematically reinforced by reward (a token) that could be exchanged for some other more tangible reward such as cigarettes or sweets.

The two theories that led to developments are classical and operant conditioning learning and are described below.

Classical and operant learning theories

Classical conditioning theory is based on the work of Pavlov, a Russian scientist who conducted several experiments with dogs. In these experiments, the sound of a bell produced a salivatory response in dogs by pairing the sound of a bell and the presentation of food. Before the experiment, the sound of a bell would not have produced a salivatory response. This paradigm was used to explain the development of feared responses, particularly phobic states. In classical conditioning any stimulus when associated (or paired) with a situation that would usually elicit a feared response, will then trigger a feared response in itself. Figure 1.1 illustrates the classical conditioning paradigm.

In instrumental or operant conditioning (Skinner 1953), behaviour will be more likely to occur if it has been persistently rewarded. Behaviour will be less likely to be repeated if it has had unpleasant or negative consequences. Behaviour is influenced by reinforcers that can be positive (rewarding) or negative (unpleasant). A positive reinforcer might be, for example, tasty food, money, a compliment, or praise. A

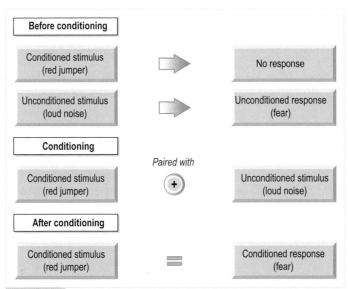

Figure 1.1 ● Classical conditioning of a fear response.

Table 1.1 • Effect of positive and negative reinforcers on behaviour

	Type of reinforcer	
	Positive	**Negative**
Reinforcer present	Increase in frequency of behaviour	Decrease in frequency of behaviour
If reinforcer **not** present	Behaviour will decrease in frequency as positive consequences do not occur	Behaviour will increase in frequency as negative consequences do not occur

negative reinforcer might be, for example, something with a sour taste, anxiety or some form of punishment.

Table 1.1 illustrates how behaviour is reinforced in operant conditioning. In operant conditioning, a feared response, such as avoidance, will be reinforced as it reduces anxiety. If avoidance is repeated, and as a consequence anxiety is repeatedly reduced, the learnt behaviour becomes established. In behaviour therapy, the feared response has to be 'unlearnt'.

Although early behaviour therapy applied learning theory and conditioning to patients' problems, its origins were in the laboratory with animal research. Only observable phenomena were considered important in understanding behaviour. Thoughts and emotions were considered as unnecessary to understanding behaviour. Behaviour therapists themselves began to revise their models and included a role for cognitive factors in understanding behaviour (Homme 1965). Around the same time as Beck was observing patients and developing his cognitive theory of emotional disorders, Albert Ellis was developing rational emotive therapy (RET), a therapy that corrects faulty thinking and processing of information to maximize rational thinking (Ellis 1962). Both Beck and Ellis included behavioural exercises in their therapies in the developing cognitive therapies, thereby acknowledging the value of behaviour therapy.

Although large numbers of people began to benefit from the new behavioural therapies, particularly for anxiety states, little progress was made in the treatment of depression until the emergence of cognitive therapy (Rachman 1997). Since cognitive therapy (Beck et al 1979) was shown to be an efficacious treatment in major depression in the original trials in the 1970s (Rush et al 1977, McLean & Hakstian 1979), the therapy has been developed to treat a wide variety of mental health disorders and specific cognitive theories have been developed to account for different types of problems and disorders.

Basic assumption of cognitive therapy

Cognitive therapy is a systematic, structured psychotherapy designed to alleviate symptoms and to help patients learn more effective ways to overcome the problems and difficulties that contribute to their distress. Cognitive therapy is based on a comprehensive theory of psychopathology and the therapy is built on therapeutic techniques directly related to the model.

The basic tenet of cognitive theory is that individuals actively process information from the environment and that problems arise as a result of an individual's interpretation of a situation or event (Beck 1967). An individual's knowledge, perceptions, interpretations and memories are all products of information processing whereby environmental and other stimuli that impinge on an individual are selected, filtered and interpreted. Individuals attach meaning to events, and the meaning of the event will vary depending on how it is interpreted. An inaccurate interpretation or a highly idiosyncratic interpretation of an event or experience can lead to a maladaptive emotional and behavioural response.

When depressed, patients have a train of thought or internal monologue of which they are barely conscious. It is this stream of thought that is negatively biased and is never questioned and rarely reported in social speech. These thoughts are called 'automatic thoughts' in cognitive therapy. They are the immediate running commentary that appears to be an accurate reflection of a person's experience. In depression, these automatic thoughts are negatively biased in a highly specific way. The content of these thoughts will be negative toned and relate to self, the world around the individual, and the future. These three components have been labelled the negative cognitive triad in depression (Beck 1976) and are thought to be an integral part of the depressive syndrome (Beck 1984).

The specific content of thoughts is likely to be related to specific disorders. In anxiety disorders, the content of thought is likely to be related to personal psychological threat or danger. In depression the content of thought will be related to loss and deprivation. A consistent relationship between thoughts of loss and failure has been found and the symptoms of depression, low mood states and the diagnosis of depression, but the relationship between anxiety symptoms and thoughts of threat and danger are less clear (see Clark & Steer 1996 for a review of studies).

Cognitive model for depression

Specific cognitive models have been developed for specific disorders such as generalized anxiety, obsessive–compulsive disorder and post-traumatic stress disorder. Beck's cognitive model of depression is illustrated in Figure 1.2.

The cognitive model of depression (Beck 1967, 1976) suggests that experiences, particularly in childhood, lead individuals to develop assumptions about the world and themselves. Individuals make sense of the world around them by attending to, organizing and evaluating information. This process is both normal and essential for surviving in the world. The assumptions we hold about the world and others help to guide our responses to situations and to behave in ways that are adaptive to our surroundings. Some of the assumptions we hold, however, may not be accurate or helpful. For example, assumptions such as 'I must always put others' needs before my own if I am to be liked' or 'Others will think poorly of me if I do not succeed' may be dysfunctional attitudes. Difficulties can occur if a situation arises that is directly linked with an individual's set of beliefs or assumptions. For example, not gaining promotion, or being ignored or not appreciated by others, could lead to an individual

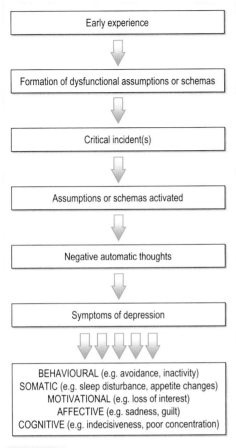

Figure 1.2 ● The cognitive model of depression.

thinking that he was not worthy of success or not liked and this in turn could lead to unhappiness and depression.

From the model of depression, it can be seen that once a dysfunctional assumption is activated, negative automatic thoughts increase. These negative automatic thoughts will be related to the underlying assumptions in content, and will also relate to the immediate situation. These negative automatic thoughts are associated with negative emotions such as depressed affect and anxiety. The symptoms of depression are related to the automatic thoughts.

Like cognitive models for other disorders, the cognitive model for depression emphasizes that informational processing is dysfunctional. The way in which information is perceived and processed not only leads to depression but also maintains depressed affect and behaviour. Three types of cognitive variables are recognized: content of thought, cognitive processing and schemata.

Content of thought

Negative view of self. When listening to a depressed patient talking, a clinician will be aware that the content of a patient's thoughts are negative. He will regard himself in negative light and describe himself in a self-derogatory manner. He will think that he is stupid, useless, and incapable of doing things and that he is unworthy.

Negative view of the world. This same patient will describe being overwhelmed by problems and unable to think of possible solutions to his problems. He may feel that his situation is frustrating and unrewarding and that there is no possibility that the situation will change. Events that happen in the world around him, even though they have no direct bearing on him, may also be viewed as examples of how difficult and obstructive the world in general has become.

Negative view of the future. As he looks to the future, this patient can only envisage that his problems will continue or may even get worse. He feels hopeless and unable to help himself as he feels overwhelmed, or lacking the necessary resources to make changes.

These three aspects of thinking in depression have been labelled the **negative cognitive triad** by Beck (1976). There is a reciprocal relationship between the content of the thoughts in the negative cognitive triad and the symptoms of depression. For example, a negative view of self would lead to, or maintain, symptoms of sadness, lack of confidence, indecisiveness and lack of motivation and inactivity. Likewise, the experience of these symptoms would be likely to lead to, or maintain, a negative view of self. A negative view of the future could lead to increasing hopelessness and this in turn could lead to an individual contemplating suicide. It is probably less clear how the more biological symptoms of depression such as loss of appetite, libido and sleep disturbance directly relate to the cognitive triad other than through a more complex relationship between thinking and biochemical and physiological events with each having an influence on the other (see Chapter 3 for a fuller discussion).

8

Cognitive processing

The content of the negative automatic thoughts of depressed patients is biased in specific ways. Five types of errors have been identified as being characteristic of information processing in depression. Blackburn & Eunson (1988) analysed the content of 50 depressed patients' thoughts and found that the errors shown in Table 1.2 accounted for the cognitive processes in depression. Some thoughts can be classified under more than one type of error. The most common error is selective abstraction.

Schemata

These are stable knowledge structures representing all the knowledge an individual has of self and the world. As seen in the cognitive model of depression, an individual's earlier experiences may contribute to a vulnerability to depression that is triggered by a stressful life event. Depressogenic schemas will usually be concerned with themes of loss, worthlessness, defeat and deprivation. When activated these depressogenic schemas will bias and distort information, and as a consequence, will lead to other symptoms of depression. Beck (1967) considered the activation of the schemas as being the mechanism by which depression develops, though the cause of depression may be multifaceted and include biological, developmental, environmental genetic and cognitive factors.

Table 1.2 ● Examples of thinking errors

Type of information processing error	Example of situation and negative automatic thought
Selective abstraction: Selecting one aspect of a situation and interpreting the whole situation on the basis of this one detail	*Situation:* Friends coming for a meal. Main course is an hour late as 'somebody' turned oven off *Thought:* 'I am a really disorganized, incompetent person. The whole evening is ruined'
Arbitrary inference: Reaching a conclusion without enough evidence to support that conclusion	*Situation:* Colleagues Sarah and John go into John's room and close door behind them *Thought:* 'They are going to talk about me'
Overgeneralization: Drawing a general conclusion on the basis of one aspect of the situation which has been arbitrarily selected from the whole context	*Situation:* Colleagues Sarah and John go into John's room and close door behind them *Thought:* 'Everyone in the department must be talking about me'
Magnification and minimization: Exaggerating the negative aspects of a situation and minimizing a positive aspect	*Situation:* Friends round for a meal and main course is an hour late *Thought:* 'All the food was terrible. The whole meal was ruined'
Personalization: Relating external events to oneself when there is no basis for making such a connection	*Situation:* Friends leave party early *Thought:* 'They thought the party was boring'

Main characteristics of cognitive–behavioural therapy

Cognitive therapy is a structured, short-term therapy based on a thorough understanding of the specific disorder being treated and how the disorder has affected the patient. Therapists need to have in-depth knowledge of the disorder being treated and need to have basic skills in interviewing so that important and relevant symptoms and problems can be elicited from the patients. Therapists should convey to their patients that they have understood their problems and should be able to formulate the patients' problems within the cognitive therapy framework.

Time limited

The therapy is time limited and comparatively brief. In routine clinical work with a depressed patient, experienced therapists will probably treat an individual for around 4 months during which they may have had around 10 to 16 appointments.

The length of therapy will of course vary depending on the disorder being treated, with some problems, such as panic attacks, requiring much briefer treatment and others, such as personality disorders, requiring longer treatment. Each session tends to last 1 hour and is structured to maximize the use of time and to target relevant problems.

Follows an agreed agenda

Cognitive therapists set an agenda with each patient. Each session therefore begins with a brief outline of how the session will be structured, taking into account progress with presenting problems, a review of homework and comments from the previous session. The agenda helps to keep the therapy structured and is agreed by both patient and therapist. Each problem is assessed and is defined precisely. This clarity is important as therapy aims to ameliorate the presenting problems and these are reviewed regularly and form the main focus of all sessions. On the whole, cognitive therapy deals with the here and now and is ahistorical.

Guided discovery

One of the main characteristics of cognitive–behavioural therapy is the type of questions that are asked to elucidate and explore problems. This type of questioning has been called guided discovery. This is a series of questions designed to bring into the patient's awareness feelings and automatic thoughts and to facilitate the promotion of alternative ways of thinking about problems and issues so that distress associated with the problem can be modified. A scientific method is used to assess and evaluate progress with problem resolution.

Experiments and homework

Patients and therapists generate hypotheses to account for the maintenance of problems. From these hypotheses, experiments are devised and carried out and the results evaluated to find out if the problem has ameliorated. Often these quasi-experiments are carried out as homework tasks. Homework tasks are designed for several purposes, such as collecting data about problems, experimenting with changes in behaviour (experiments), and practising cognitive techniques to capture and modify automatic thoughts and beliefs.

Cognitive formulation

The patient's problems are described in a cognitive formulation – a working hypothesis that ties together the problems, thoughts and feelings and hypothesized underlying beliefs within the cognitive model. Therapists should be able from the formulation to provide a possible explanation as to why problems may have arisen and are maintained. Although the main work of therapy is largely ahistorical, the formulation is likely to use historical data gathered during the assessment period of therapy. The formulation should be shared with the patient to aid collaboration and understanding.

Specific therapeutic techniques

Specific cognitive and behavioural techniques will vary according to the problem or disorder being treated and the specific problems that the patient presents in therapy. Chapters on specific problems or disorders are included in this book, illustrating how cognitive therapy and the cognitive model have been adapted.

The empirical basis of cognitive–behavioural therapy

Cognitive–behavioural therapy (CBT) was one of the first psychological therapies to be systematically assessed in terms of treatment outcome. A body of scientific literature spanning over 30 years now exists that examines the impact of CBT on a variety of major mental disorders and other problems. Butler et al (2006) found a total of 16 methodologically rigorous meta-analyses for CBT with outcomes for various control groups for a variety of disorders. Large effect sizes were found for CBT for unipolar depression, generalized anxiety disorder, panic disorder with or without agoraphobia, social phobia, post-traumatic stress disorder, and childhood depressive and anxiety disorders. Effect sizes for CBT of marital distress, anger, childhood somatic disorders, and chronic pain were in the moderate range. CBT was equally effective as behaviour therapy in the treatment of adult depression and obsessive–compulsive disorder. CBT was somewhat superior to antidepressants in the treatment of adult depression. In a review of studies of CBT in depression, Gloaguen et al (1998) found that CBT was significantly better than antidepressant medication. However, this conclusion may overstate the case for CBT since this review included some early studies comparing CBT with medications which had methodological features that favoured CBT. A more recent high-quality controlled trial comparing CBT with a commonly prescribed serotonin reuptake inhibitor, paroxetine, found that cognitive therapy was equally effective for the initial treatment of moderate to severe major depression (Hollon et al 2005). Other therapies have also been shown to be effective in the treatment of major depression such as interpersonal psychotherapy (IPT). The Treatment of Depression Collaborative Research Project (TDCRP) compared the efficacy of CBT, interpersonal psychotherapy and pharmacotherapy for depression. Outcomes for CBT and interpersonal therapy were found to be almost equivalent (Elkin et al 1989) but CBT did not fare as well as IPT or antidepressant medication among those patients with more severe depression.

Developments in cognitive–behavioural therapy in mental health

Metacognition and cognitive therapy

As stated earlier, in Beck's original model of emotions (Beck 1976), negative thoughts and interpretations are thought to arise from the activation of dysfunctional schemas. Once activated, dysfunctional schemas introduce biases in the way information is processed and interpreted, thereby maintaining depression. This schema model gives us an explanation of why the content of thinking in depression is negative but does not tell us the reason for this particular style of thinking.

Wells & Matthews (1994, 1996) propose that the style of thinking is a key factor in psychological disorders. In their model, they link schema theory with information processing and self-regulation and suggest that the metacognitive level of belief is important in regulating the self. Three levels of architecture are proposed that support information processing operations. At low-level processing, most information processing is automatic and is outside conscious awareness. At an intermediate level, there is controlled processing whereby an individual makes conscious appraisals of events and has control of thoughts and actions. At the highest level, there is self-knowledge, or beliefs, stored in long-term memory. Each level interacts with the level immediately above or below. These three levels are thought to represent the total range of processing operations available to an individual, but different modes and processing configurations are possible. For the main part, appraisals of stimuli, thoughts and perceptions are regarded as being accurate representations. However, in a metacognitive mode, thoughts and perceptions are not necessarily accepted as being accurate representations of reality. In the latter mode, an individual can have distance from his or her own thoughts and perceptions and therefore can evaluate them.

They propose that in psychological disorders, problems arise with self-relevant information processing and self-regulation. Self-regulatory executive functioning focuses attention on the self, and appraises the personal significance of external events as well as the body state and cognitive response (Wells 2000). Ideally, an individual will be able to self-regulate by appraising information and selecting coping strategies, either behavioural or cognitive, which are appropriate to achieving a desired goal or normative state. Self-regulatory executive functioning activity is usually short-lived and appraisals are accepted as being accurate representation of reality. However, Wells (2000) argues that in psychological disorders, a person is unable to achieve self-regulatory goals as the pattern of cognitive processing activated becomes dysfunctional.

Implications for metacognitive model for treatment

The self-regulatory executive functioning model may allow cognitive therapy to develop some new approaches to treating emotional disorders. In particular, it may be particularly helpful in the treatment of disorders such as obsessive–compulsive disorder (OCD) and generalized anxiety disorder where the style of dysfunctional processing is more metacognitive. Individuals with obsessive–compulsive disorder experience recurrent unwanted intrusive ruminations and compulsions. Some individuals with OCD, for example, believe that if they think about something bad happening, it will happen. This is known as thought–event fusion (Wells 1997). Metacognitive awareness and strategies may be able to modify these types of problems.

In conventional therapy for OCD, the goal of therapy would be to stop obsessive thinking and behavioural rituals. The goal in therapy using a metacognitive model would be to recognize that beliefs about thinking in particular ways were not necessarily accurate and that they need not be acted upon. By becoming more aware of the type of thinking pattern, a distinction is made between a thought and a fact, and a thought and an action. Both distinctions would be helpful in breaking the link between compulsive thoughts and ritualistic behaviours and help the individual to stand back and distance himself from his thoughts.

Cognitive–behavioural therapy for psychotic disorder

In the past decade there has been increasing interest in cognitive–behavioural interventions for those with schizophrenia, and reviews of the research literature would suggest that the findings are positive for reducing residual positive and negative symptoms at the end of therapy (Rector & Beck 2001, Pilling et al 2002). Over 20 randomized controlled trials have been published, the majority of these concerned with alleviating medication resistant symptoms in chronic patients, but some preliminary work has also been carried out with speeding recovery in acute phases of schizophrenia and in relapse prevention and early intervention. A review of these studies indicates modest effect sizes, with the strongest evidence available for chronic patients (Tarrier & Wykes 2004).

Generally these interventions have focused on reducing distress and the disabling effect of psychotic symptoms as well as improving mood and reducing social disability. Attempts at recognizing and reducing signs indicative of relapse have also been made. It has been found that readiness to consider an alternative explanation for delusions was a predictor of good outcome for those with a psychotic disorder who had at least one distressing, treatment-resistant positive psychotic symptom (such as delusions or hallucinations) treated with cognitive therapy (Garety et al 1997, Kuipers et al 1997).

Interventions are based on the idea that positive symptoms such as delusions, that are part of the diagnosis of schizophrenia, can be regarded as abnormal beliefs. As such, these beliefs can be thought of as arising as a consequence of perceptual or reasoning deficits (Hemsley & Garety 1986) and cause an individual to misconstrue or misunderstand what is happening in reality. Other psychological models of delusions have emphasized the role of attributional bias in the formation of persecutory delusions (Bentall et al 2001). In this latter model, attributions made about the cause of events are thought to influence self-representations and this, in turn, influences other attributions. Negative events are regarded as being caused by external agents and this attribution creates a more paranoid view of the world (see Chapter 6 for fuller discussion).

Personality disorder

Personality disorders are characterized by long-standing and pervasive dysfunctional patterns of cognitive, affect, interpersonal relationships and impulse control (DSM-IV; American Psychiatric Association 1994). These dysfunctional patterns cause considerable distress and impairment in psychosocial functioning and those individuals with personality disorder, particularly those who deliberately self-harm, tend to be heavy users of health services (Rissmiller et al 1994, Rodger & Scott 1995). Although there are ten types of personality disorders in the current American diagnostic system (DSM-IV), borderline personality disorders are probably among the

13

most frequently found types of personality disorder found in the Health Service, partly as a result of individuals with this diagnosis self-harming and from actively seeking help for problems (American Psychiatric Association 1994).

The cognitive theory of personality disorder is essentially a biosocial theory that proposes that there is an exaggeration of pre-programmed patterns of behaviour that through evolution promoted individual survival and reproduction in personality disorder (Beck et al 1990). These patterns of behaviour or strategies are related to underlying cognitive, affective and motivational patterns or schemas that affect the way information about self or the environment is processed. Cognitive therapy for borderline personality disorder (Davidson 2007) has been adapted to resolve the long-standing problems found in personality disorder. Compared to cognitive therapy for other disorders, there is more emphasis on childhood and adolescent experiences in cognitive therapy for personality disorder. The focus of therapy is at the level of core beliefs rather than on automatic thoughts. Further differences emerge in the modification of beliefs and behaviours. In other disorders, the emphasis is on modifying thinking and behaviour and patients have the experience of behaving in more flexible ways and, even if currently suffering from a disorder, have personal experiences and memories of more adaptive behaviour and thinking when healthy. In cognitive therapy of personality disorders, the beliefs are long-standing, rigidly held and may to some extent make sense of dysfunctional relationships in childhood. The behaviour patterns are similarly pervasive, rigid and inflexible. To develop more adaptive, flexible thinking and behaviour, cognitive therapy for personality disorders requires patients to develop new thinking and behaviour.

There is some evidence that psychotherapy is effective in the treatment of a number of different types of personality disorders, particularly psychodynamic and cognitive–behavioural therapies (Leichsenring & Leibing 2003) though the majority of studies have not been randomized controlled trials. Recent evidence from a randomized controlled trial suggests that CBT may be effective in the treatment of borderline personality disorder, reducing suicidal acts, distress, and dysfunctional beliefs compared to usual treatment (Davidson et al 2006, Giesen-Bloo et al 2006).

Common myths about cognitive–behavioural therapy

In cognitive–behavioural therapy, therapists have to correct the patient's thinking

In the emotional disorders, thinking is biased in specific ways. This does not imply that the patient's thinking is wrong but suggests that they are processing information in an unhelpful, skewed manner. Cognitive–behavioural therapy aims to help the patient identify the types of thinking biases experienced during an episode of illness. Once identified, the patient can then learn to systematically challenge the specific content of thought so that a less biased, more realistic judgement of a situation or experience can be ascertained.

Cognitive–behavioural therapy is just a collection of techniques

The techniques used in cognitive–behavioural therapy are powerful in changing thinking, emotions and behaviour. If however, these techniques are not applied within a cognitive framework or formulation, they are likely to be less helpful to the patient. Patients and therapists need to have a clear idea of the rationale for using specific techniques.

Therapists have to work at the level of dysfunctional assumptions, not automatic thoughts

For many problems, working at the level of automatic thoughts is sufficiently powerful to ameliorate most distressing symptoms and help the patient to get better. Working at the level of dysfunctional assumptions may, however, increase the patient's understanding of the problems experienced and may help the patient to develop more helpful beliefs in the longer-term.

Cognitive–behavioural therapy does not take into consideration the therapeutic relationship

Unlike some other forms of psychotherapy, cognitive–behavioural therapy has not developed a systematic agreed language to describe the therapeutic relationship. Nonetheless, in practice, cognitive–behavioural therapy does take the therapeutic relationship into account. This is best described as forming a collaborative relationship with the patient. The characteristics of the collaboration are that the relationship is professional, open and working on the presenting problems. It is likely, however, that more emphasis will be placed on describing the parameters of the therapeutic relationship in the future as cognitive–behavioural therapy is increasingly used with individuals who have significant interpersonal difficulties that are also likely to impede progress in therapy.

It does not matter if my patient does not carry out homework assignments

Many cognitive–behavioural therapists find that patients are not always compliant with homework assignments. However, compliance does seem to improve outcomes. As such, it is worthwhile paying particular attention to making the homework tasks relevant and achievable.

All health professionals would benefit from learning about cognitive–behavioural therapy

Given that cognitive therapy epitomizes evidence-based treatment, is acceptable to patients and can be readily understood, it would be worthwhile learning at least something about cognitive–behavioural therapies. Although becoming an expert in the area takes time and effort to develop the necessary skills, becoming familiar with the cognitive–behavioural model will give a psychological framework to understand and communicate to others about problems. This psychological framework emphasizes the importance of understanding the nature of faulty information processing on mood, emotions and behaviour and the impact this has on an individual's emotional and physical well-being.

References

American Psychiatric Association 1994 Diagnostic and statistical manual of mental disorders, 4th edn. Washington, DC

Beck A T 1963 Thinking and depression. I. Idiosyncratic content and cognitive distortions. Archives of General Psychiatry 9:324–333

Beck A T 1967 Depression: clinical, experimental, and theoretical aspects. Hoeber, New York

Beck A T 1976 Cognitive therapy and the emotional disorders. International Universities Press, New York

Beck A T 1984 Cognition and therapy. Archives of General Psychiatry 41:1112–1114

Beck A T, Ward C H 1961 Dreams of depressed patients: characteristic themes in manifest content. Archives of General Psychiatry 5:462–467

Beck A T, Rush A J, Shaw B F et al 1979 Cognitive therapy of depression: a treatment manual. Guilford Press, New York

Beck A T, Freeman A & Associates 1990 Cognitive therapy of personality disorders. Guilford Press, New York

Bentall R P, Corcoran R, Howard R et al 2001 Persecutory delusions: a review and theoretical integration. Clinical Psychology Review 21(8):1143–1192

Blackburn I M, Eunson K M 1988 A content analysis of thoughts and emotions elicited from depressed patients during cognitive therapy. British Journal of Medical Psychology 62:23–33

Butler A C, Chapman J E, Forman E M et al 2006 The empirical status of cognitive-behavioral therapy: a review of meta-analyses. Clinical Psychology Review Ch 26, pp 17–31

Clark D A, Steer R A 1996 Empirical status of the cognitive model of anxiety and depression. In: Salkovskis P M (ed) Frontiers of cognitive therapy. Guilford Press, New York

Davidson K M 2007 Cognitive therapy for personality disorders: a guide for clinicians, 2nd edn. Routledge, Hove

Davidson K, Norrie J, Tyrer P et al 2006 The effectiveness of cognitive behaviour therapy for borderline personality disorder: results from the BOSCOT trial. Journal of Personality Disorders 20:450–465

Elkin I, Shea M, Watkins S et al 1989 National institute of mental health treatment of depression collaborative research program: general effectiveness of treatments. Archives of General Psychiatry 46: 971–982

Ellis A 1962 Reason and emotion in psychotherapy. Lynne Stuart, Seacausus, NJ

Garety P, Fowler D, Kuipers E et al 1997 London–East Anglia randomised controlled trial of cognitive–behavioural therapy for psychosis. II: Predictors of outcome. British Journal of Psychiatry 171:420–426

Giesen-Bloo J, van Dyck R, Spinhoven P et al 2006 Outpatient psychotherapy for borderline personality disorder: randomized trial of schema-focused therapy vs transference-focused psychotherapy. Archives of General Psychiatry 63: 649–658

Gloaguen V, Cottraux J, Cucherat M et al 1998 A meta-analysis of the effects of cognitive therapy in depressed patients. Journal of Affective Disorders 49:59–72

Hemsley D R, Garety P A 1986 The formation and maintenance of delusions: a Bayesian analysis. British Journal of Psychiatry 149:51–56

Hollon S D, DeRubeis R J, Shelton R C et al 2005 Prevention of relapse following cognitive therapy vs medications in moderate to severe depression. Archives of General Psychiatry 62:417–422

Homme L E 1965 Perspectives in psychology: XXIV control of coverants; the operants of the mind. Psychological Record 15:501–511

Kuipers E, Garety P A, Fowler D et al 1997 The London–East Anglia trial of cognitive behaviour therapy for psychosis I: effects of the treatment phase. British Journal of Psychiatry 171:319–327

Leichsenring F, Leibing E 2003 The effectiveness of psychodynamic therapy and cognitive behavior therapy in the treatment of personality disorders: a meta-analysis. American Journal of Psychiatry 160:1223–1232

McLean P D, Hakstian A R 1979 Clinical depression: comparative efficacy of out-patient treatments. Journal of Consulting and Clinical Psychology 47:818–836

Pilling S, Bebbington P, Kuipers E et al 2002 Psychological treatments in schizophrenia I: meta-analysis of family intervention and cognitive behavioural therapy. Psychological Medicine 32:63–782

Rachman S. 1997 The evolution of cognitive behaviour therapy. In: Clark D M, Fairburn C G (eds) Science and practice of cognitive behaviour therapy. Oxford Medical Publications, Oxford

Rector N, Beck A T 2001 Cognitive behavioural therapy for schizophrenia: an empirical review. Journal of Nervous and Mental Disease 189:278–287

Rissmiller D J, Steer R, Ranieri W F et al 1994 Factors complicating cost containment in the treatment of suicidal patients. Hospital Community Psychiatry 45:782–788

Rodger C R, Scott A I 1995 Frequent deliberate self-harm: repetition, suicide and cost after three or more years. Journal of Scottish Medicine 40:10–12

Rush A J, Beck A T, Kovacs M et al 1977 Comparative efficacy of cognitive therapy versus pharmacotherapy in out-patient depression. Cognitive Therapy and Research 1:17–37

Skinner B F 1953 Science and human behaviour. Macmillan, New York

Tarrier N, Wykes T 2004 Is there evidence that cognitive behaviour therapy is an effective treatment for schizophrenia? A cautious or cautionary tale? Behaviour Research and Therapy 42: 1377–1401

Weishaar M E 1993 Aaron T. Beck. Key figures in Counselling and psychotherapy. Sage Publications, London

Wells A 1997 Cognitive therapy of anxiety disorders: a practice manual and conceptual guide. John Wiley, Chichester

Wells A 2000 Emotional disorders and meta-cognition, John Wiley, Chichester

Wells A, Matthews G 1994 Attention and emotion: a clinical perspective. Erlbaum, Hove

Wells A, Matthews G 1996 Modelling cognition in emotional disorder: the S-REF model. Behaviour Research and Therapy 32:867–870

Incorporating cognitive–behavioural approaches into models of practice

Maggie Nicol

Introduction

The authors of this book firmly believe that to enhance the professions of occupational therapy and physiotherapy there needs to be strong theoretical underpinning to practice, associated with relevant assessments and intervention strategies which can be subject to evaluation, thus strengthening the evidence base of both professions. This chapter will briefly explore the terminology and concepts associated with models of practice, then discuss two models of practice commonly used, the model of human occupation (MOHO), a unidisciplinary model, and biopsychosocial, a multi-disciplinary model. Cognitive–behavioural techniques will be linked to both models to demonstrate that models of practice should not be viewed as static but dynamic tools which can incorporate appropriate interventions from other areas where evidence of their effectiveness has been demonstrated.

What is a model of practice?

When exploring the literature concerning models of practice there is little agreement about the terminology used. The terms theory, paradigm, model, frame of reference and approach have all been defined and used. Kortman (1995) in analysing the use of the terms suggests that theorists are taking the wrong path in trying to constantly define terms. He maintains that the terms are interchangeable and that the term model is the simplest to use. For readers who wish to explore this issue in more depth Hagedorn (1997) offers two useful tables, which identify the terminology used by American and British occupational therapists to describe theory. Kielhofner (1995, p 13) advocates for the term conceptual models of practice, as 'it is no longer advisable to separate the search for knowledge from the search for solving problems'. He proposes that conceptual models of practice aim to:

it presents. It guides the activity and occupational choices that together determine much of what we do . . . To a large extent, how we experience life and how we regard ourselves and our world has to do with volition' (Kielhofner 2002, p 59).

Kielhofner (2002, p 14) argues that humans have a 'biological mandate to be active', but that in itself is not enough to explain why we choose certain occupations. He maintains that in addition to the biological need for activity other factors are involved in motivation. Specifically, choices to engage in occupations are mediated by thoughts and feelings related to personal effectiveness, worth or importance of the occupation and enjoyment experienced when undertaking the occupation. These three concepts he labelled personal causation, values and interests.

Personal causation

Personal causation focuses on how competent and effective we perceive ourselves to be in certain occupations along with the feelings that attend these perceptions. We develop our concept of our competence and effectiveness based on:

- an assessment of our physical, intellectual and social capabilities which within the model is called sense of personal capacity

combined with

- how we feel our effectiveness is when achieving desired outcomes in day-to-day life which is labelled within this model as self-efficacy.

Many of the individuals whom occupational therapists and physiotherapists work with have a negative sense of capacity and self-efficacy. We often have clients tell us 'I can't do that' and will be reluctant to attempt new challenges. Many occupational therapists and physiotherapists spend considerable time within the therapy context challenging these negative views while persuading clients to attempt new challenges and have experienced the delight of the person when they achieve success.

Values

From the earliest point in our lives we develop views about the things that matter to us and over our lifespan we learn to appreciate what is good, right and important. Kielhofner (2002, p 50) suggests, 'values commit us to a way of life and impart commonsense meaning to the lives we lead'. Values, within MOHO, are conceptualized into two areas, personal convictions and a sense of obligation. Personal convictions tend to be shaped by 'a view of how the world is and the identification of what matters' (Kielhofner 2002, p 51). Personal convictions vary from individual to individual but tend to shape the life we lead.

Sense of obligation refers to the feelings and behaviour which induce us to act in the right way according to our values.

Many occupational therapists and physiotherapists see clients who have experienced disability and who can no longer live up to their values. These clients often experience a loss of self-worth and question their existence.

Interests

We develop our interest from the enjoyment we experience when carrying out activities, which leads us to be attracted to certain types of activities. This helps us understand why, for instance, some people are attracted to the outdoor sporting life while others favour more sedentary, indoor occupations. We each tend to develop a unique interest pattern of occupations which we prefer to engage in which give us satisfaction and enjoyment.

Occupational therapists and physiotherapists often meet clients whose interest pattern has been either disrupted or limited because of disability or illness and this often has a profound affect on their satisfaction with life.

Habituation

For people to function in life they tend to have internal information which results in recurring patterns of behaviour which allow them to go about their everyday life. This allows us to repeat our usual daily routines without consciously thinking about what we are doing. This semi-autonomous process within MOHO is referred to as habituation. To behave in a consistent routine within our usual physical, social and cultural environments we tend to utilize habits and roles.

Habits

We tend to develop habits by repeating actions in the same way in the same setting at the same time and once acquired they tend to become automatic. Habits help shape and structure our daily life. Habits are therefore within MOHO defined as 'acquired tendencies to automatically respond and perform in certain, consistent ways in familiar environments or situations' (Kielhofner 2002, p 65).

Habits can become disrupted or eroded due to illness or disability and this can have a major impact on the individual's lifestyle. Often occupational therapists and physiotherapist in partnership with the client are instrumental in helping re-establish or develop new habit patterns.

Roles

All of us have roles which allow us to define ourselves within society or person-ally, each of these roles carries with it expectations, responsibilities, privileges and expected behaviour associated with the role. People tend to know how to behave in a role because they have an internalized role script which they have learned which enables them to perform when in that role. Additionally, roles tend to support a person's self-identity. Roles can change over the lifespan.

People who have or develop illnesses or disabilities may have roles removed or changed and barriers to adopting new roles may be imposed. Occupational thera-pists and physiotherapist often act as advocates for clients in helping them develop current or new challenging roles.

When habituation is affected, individuals lose a sense of the familiar and routine, as we require habits and roles to function effectively within society.

Performance capacity

The ability to engage in occupations depends on a complex interaction between the mind and body. We need our physical, cognitive and social capabilities to suc-cessfully perform occupations. Many existing models used by occupational thera-pists and physiotherapists focus specifically at the objective physical and mental

23

components. Loss of function is understood in terms of impairments in any of the physical or mental systems.

Occupational capacity within MOHO includes these concepts but also extends beyond this and is defined as 'the ability for doing things provided by the status of underlying objective physical and mental components and corresponding subjective experience' (Kielhofner 2002, p 25). The concept of subjective experience is explained by the term 'lived body'. Within MOHO this is defined as 'experience of being and knowing the world through a particular body' (Kielhofner 2002, p 83). This relates not to the physical/mental capacities which are required to do the occupation but to what it feels like to do the occupation. The concept of the lived body is a developing one and Kielhofner (2002) illustrates this in his textbook with three clinical studies which describe this concept.

Environment

Individuals do not exist in a vacuum and the role of the environment is considered within MOHO. The environment within MOHO covers the physical, social and cultural and specifically considers the environmental role affecting engaging in occupations. MOHO is concerned with the opportunities, resources, demands and constraints which the environment places on individuals.

Occupational therapists and physiotherapists have experienced many examples from clients which demonstrate the positive or negative effect the environment in its totality can have on the lives of people with disabilities.

All of the aspects above come together in the concepts of occupational identity and occupational competence. Occupational identity is 'composite sense of who one is and wishes to become as an occupational being generated from one's history of occupational participation', while occupational competence is 'the degree to which one is able to sustain a pattern of occupational participation that reflects one's occupational identity' (Kielhofner 2002, p 122). Both of these develop as we engage in occupations but we need to have an occupational identity which we can then put into action. Illness and disability can impact on both of these concepts resulting in a poor or diminished occupational identity which results in failure to engage in occupations or occupational identity remains but the ability to enact it is impaired.

MOHO in practice

As already highlighted in an earlier section there needs to be more to models of practice than theoretical understanding. Models of practice must have methods of assessment and intervention strategies to allow for their use in practice. Several assessments are available to assess aspects of the individual based on a theoretical understanding of the MOHO framework. These assessments, which have undergone rigorous testing and development, evaluate individual aspects of MOHO, e.g. Role Checklist which looks specifically at role; other assessments assess all aspects of MOHO, e.g. Occupational Performance History Interview (OPHI).

For further detailed descriptions of all these assessments readers should consult Kielhofner (2002) and the website mentioned above. Most of the assessments can be obtained directly from the website.

Having gathered client data the next stage is to establish with the client what the areas of concern and competencies are and to prioritize these into intervention strategies to facilitate change in the client.

MOHO has identified the following range of client actions which occur during therapy:

- Commit to a course of action
- Explore new ways of carrying out actions
- Identify new information, ideas or feelings
- Negotiate an agreed upon plan of action
- Plan an agenda for action
- Practice appropriate actions/occupations/skills
- Re-examine beliefs, attitudes, habits or roles
- Sustain effort over time

One of the main strategies within MOHO is for the therapist to support and enable the client's engagement in occupation. In order to provide this support the following strategies have been identified:

- Validate the client's experiences
- Identify clients' potential actions which will encourage engagement in occupations
- Give feedback to the client
- Advise the client about intervention strategies
- Negotiate with clients
- Structure the client's engagement in occupations
- Coach client in appropriate ways
- Encourage clients
- Provide physical support

Within the most recent edition of the Model of Human Occupation a helpful master table is presented which provides guidelines for client engagement and therapists' strategies based on the concepts of the model.

As this brief discussion of MOHO should make obvious, this model shares a number of features with cognitive–behavioural therapy (CBT). Like CBT it sees emotions, cognition and behaviour as linked, emphasizing the modifiability of these three elements. MOHO focuses on this through the use of occupation by identifying meaning, habits and skill, whereas CBT has been used to understand maladaptive thinking, behaviour and emotion in the context of distress. In this regard it is a helpful complement to the CBT approach. Taylor (2005) argues that MOHO is an important complement to CBT since the former provides well-developed conceptualization and practice strategies surrounding the volition and lifestyle and performance capacity.

Case Study 2.1 highlights how MOHO and cognitive–behavioural techniques can be combined.

CASE STUDY 2.1

Jack is 35 years old and has had mental health problems for many years resulting in many in-patient admissions and finally, following a serious assault, a period in a medium secure unit where he is currently being treated.

The occupational therapist was keen to understand Jack as an individual and learn what his needs, wishes and experiences were. MOHO assessments focus primarily on occupational life rather than symptoms and diagnosis and therefore are a useful vehicle to learn about Jack and to develop trust. In considering the appropriate assessment tools to use from the array available the occupational therapists knew Jack was articulate and could tell his story so she chose the Occupational Performance History Interview second version (OPHIE-11) as an assessment tool. This allows the person to relate a detailed account of their life.

This identified that Jack entered mental health services at 19 when he dropped out of university and was diagnosed with schizophrenia. Over the intervening years he had drifted in and out of casual employment and had short periods of hospitalization when he stopped taking his medication. He has a supportive family, whom he lived with periodically when he felt he needed extra support. He had dropped out of the mental health support mechanisms and was living a fairly isolated life. The current in-patient stay occurred following an incident in a pub when Jack became violent and attacked the man standing next to him. Jack was found to be deluded and hallucinating and was admitted under the Mental Health Act to a medium secure unit. Jack has had his medication reviewed and his psychotic symptoms are no longer problematic. The following, using MOHO constructs, were identified during the interview.

Volition

Jack demonstrated that he had some positive ideas about himself, which had been bolstered by having a short story published recently. He was beginning to feel that his life might now have some meaning and success but he expressed concerns about whether he would be able to achieve his aspiration to become a writer. He identified two interests: reading literature and writing.

Habituation

Jack had a few roles he could identify and strongly valued several of them. The main one was family member but he was excited by the new role which was just emerging, that of writer. He was able to describe a habit pattern which was blighted by his psychotic symptoms and his anxiety but which mainly focused around visiting his family, reading and writing. His self-care was adequate and he expressed no concerns about this.

Performance capacity

Jack mainly reported that he was physically able to do all the things he wanted to do but that his anxiety limited his performance.

Jack was now actively talking about his wish to participate in a planned transfer within the hospital to less secure accommodation before discharge back into the local community. In order to facilitate this the following goals were agreed with Jack:

- Reduce anxiety and fear of failure in occupational performance
- Further increase sense of self-efficacy
- Increase participation in things which interest him
- Commit to enhancing roles, particularly his role as a writer

Jack identified several activities which he wanted to engage in (occupational focus):

- Visit the local library
- Join a creative writing group
- Visit his family who lived nearby

Jack was very motivated to achieve his occupational goals but his high level of anxiety interfered with his ability to carry these out. So in agreement with Jack the following goal was added:

- Learn to cope with his anxiety symptoms to enhance occupational engagement in valued activities (CBT focus)

In order for Jack to control his anxiety, which would then allow him to engage in these chosen activities, a cognitive–behavioural approach was initiated within the unit. These CBT-focused sessions helped Jack understand his symptoms and develop coping strategies which utilized challenging negative thoughts, relaxation techniques and gradual desensitization. The occupational therapist discussed the symptoms of anxiety that Jack was experiencing, paying particular attention to when and where Jack experienced more anxiety. In discussion the occupational therapist noted that Jack had anxiety-provoking thoughts in situations such as going out of the hospital. For example, on leaving the hospital grounds Jack thought 'I can't cope – my heart is racing too fast and I am going to collapse'. These thoughts were accompanied with heavy sweats and feeling shaky. These thoughts were increasing Jack's anxiety and predicting that he was going to collapse and therefore reinforcing Jack's belief that leaving the hospital was dangerous for him. The occupational therapist drew the link between his thoughts, feelings and behaviour and encouraged him to keep a record of these in a dysfunctional automatic thought record. The physiotherapist taught him relaxation techniques to cope with the physical anxiety symptoms and once these were mastered the occupational therapist introduced a graded exposure programme, whereby Jack was able to increase the distance and time that he was away from the hospital, allowing him to focus on his occupational goals. Jack was able to utilize his CBT sessions to control his anxiety, which enabled him to ultimately use his local library. This allowed him to borrow books and acted as an information point on local writing groups which he could access. The occupational therapist also encouraged him to continue writing and introduced him to another client who was also interested in writing. They eventually worked as a pair to read and critically appraise each other's work. He was also able to visit his family. Jack reported feeling very positive about this control he had over his anxiety and how this enabled him to engage in the things he wanted to do. He was now planning with the occupational therapist which writing group he would approach and how he would do that. A transfer to a less secure environment within the hospital was also being initiated. Jack was expressing reservations about the transfer but was also able to articulate how positive this would be for him and how he would use the strategies he had learned to deal with the anxiety surrounding the move.

The biopsychosocial model

This model grew out of dissatisfaction with the biomedical model which had dominated medicine for many generations. The person credited with developing this model was George Engel, who first published a paper on this topic in 1977. Engel outlined a holistic alternative to combat what he thought was the important but narrow perspective of the biomedical model. The biopsychosocial model views the biological, psychological and social systems as being interrelated with the mind affecting the body and vice versa. Engel believed that:

- The biomedical material should be complemented by the patient's subjective view.
- A model should be more comprehensive than the biomedical reductionist approach.
- More power should be given to the patient in the doctor–patient relationship thus enhancing the patient's role.

In his seminal paper discussing the clinical application of the biopsychosocial model, Engel (1980) outlined his hierarchy of natural systems. He devised 15 levels of this hierarchy. These are subatomic particles, atoms, molecules, organelles, cells, tissues, organs, nervous system, person, two person, family, community, culture, society and biosphere.

Engel endorsed the view that 'different levels of the biopsychosocial hierarchy could interact but the rules of interaction might not be directly derived from the rules of the higher and lower rungs of the biopsychosocial ladder. Rather they would be considered emergent properties that would be highly dependent on the persons involved and the initial conditions with which they presented' (Borrell-Carrio et al 2004, p 577). Engel's model was important at the time as it questioned the dominance of the biomedical model. The substance of this model suggests that the patient/client should be at the centre of the intervention and that account should be taken of the psychology, biology and social systems in which the patient/client exists. Engel's, in spite of being a dominant model subscribed to by many, fails to provide detailed theoretical knowledge of the nature of the interaction of these hierarchies.

In occupational therapy and physiotherapy, like other health professions, the biomedical model is no longer seen as a sufficient model for practice and the importance of biology, psychology and social context is well recognized. Borrell-Carrio et al (2004) have recognized the importance of respecting the patient/client and the importance of the therapeutic relationship in enhancing patient care outlining seven principles termed 'biopsychosocial orientated clinical practice' in order that health-care workers would 'infuse care with greater warmth and caring' (p 581).

Since the publication of the original article and a follow-up discussing the clinical application of the model (Engel 1980) much research reinforces the value of the model and shows how the combined effect of the physical, psychological and social process have affected health outcomes. It is not the purpose of this chapter to outline all this research but some specific examples are cited to demonstrate this; in cardiac disease and chronic back pain the role of emotions and its subsequent support is well recognized (Smith & Ruiz 2002, Blumenthal et al 2002 in Suls & Rothman 2004, Cook & Hassenkamp 2000, Waddell 1987).

Although the biopsychosocial model has its champions, it also has critics, partly due to its failure to deliver research evidence that encompasses all of these spheres. Current research paradigms are unable to investigate the inter-relationship between all three levels. McLaren (1998) from a medical perspective suggests that the original Engel model only demonstrated the need for an understanding of the way the biological and non-biological interfaced in disease and illness but did not provide detailed information on how that interface worked.

However, Suls & Rothman (2004), both health psychologists, view the biopsychosocial model as a work in progress. They suggest that 'for the biopsychosocial perspective to be fully embraced, investigators need to continue transforming it from a conceptual framework into a model that specifies the linkages between the different subsystems' (p 1221).

In defence of the model, White (2005) writing from a medical perspective suggests that psychological and social factors contribution to disease is clear. For example, cancer and heart disease are the biggest killers in this country and the commonest cause is smoking. However, it is clear that the causes of smoking are multifactorial requiring interventions which reflect this complexity.

The biopsychosocial model as a named concept originated nearly three decades ago and whilst still frequently referred to by health professionals there is a need to provide a more detailed account of some of the concepts around the mind–brain interface to provide a more theoretically robust model.

CASE STUDY 2.2

Joe, aged 55, is married with two grown-up children and is employed as a middle manager in a large company. He was admitted to the stroke unit via A & E after having a stroke resulting in a right hemiplegia. He has a history of hypertension over ten years and it has been controlled by medication.

Applying a biopsychosocial perspective, the stroke created damage to several layers of the 15 natural systems described by Engel. At the *tissue level* there was a cerebral infarction which led at the *organ* level to left-hemisphere brain failure resulting in, at the *nervous system level,* right-sided weakness to the body. This was experienced at the *person level* by Joe by features of fear, anxiety and withdrawal. This reverberated in his *two person and family level* with concern and overprotectiveness and disengagement by Joe at the *community, culture and society level.* Joe received an intensive course of rehabilitation from both physiotherapists and occupational therapists, much of it aimed at the organ and nervous systems level with prevention of deformity, use of correct patterns of movement, inhibition of abnormal movements and training in functional independence tasks. Following this Joe is able to walk, and has gross motor ability in his upper limbs with some fine finger movement yet to return.

While having achieved a relatively good recovery he is still very fearful and negative about the future, worrying about having another stroke. He is reluctant to discuss return to work or to participate in any of his previous hobbies of gardening and golf. Intervention is therefore required at his person system level with the hope that changes here will result in more changes at his family/community/ society level. It was decided that adding CBT to the treatment regimen would be beneficial. The clinical psychologist who consulted for the stroke unit developed a cognitive–behavioural regimen for Joe. These sessions focused on Joe understanding the nature of stroke and developing coping strategies which utilized challenging negative thoughts, such as 'if I become more active I will put a strain on my body and have another stroke'. Joe was also taught relaxation techniques to help control his anxiety. These sessions were carried out by a nurse, occupational therapist and physiotherapist, all of whom knew Joe well, and were overseen by the clinical psychologist. Following some classroom-type sessions the staff began to combine these cognitive–behavioural approaches with practical sessions involving coping strategies and challenging his behaviour in order to become less limited in what he did. During this time Joe was encouraged to maintain a thought diary and behavioural record of achievements. Utilising CBT questioning Joe was able to recognize that his risk of having another stroke was not as high as he had previously estimated and that he would be able to incrementally increase his activity level whilst coping with the uncertainty of a recurrence of a stroke.

Joe's wife, who was also slightly overprotective, was seen and the therapy outlined to her. Her help was enlisted so when Joe displayed negative thoughts she gently encouraged him to do what he could and reminded him of what he had achieved.

Over time Joe began to view his situation in a more realistic way and began with the help of the staff and his wife to engage in more strenuous activities.

He undertook light gardening and was making plans for the summer planting demonstrating a more positive view of the future. Joe has been in touch with his employers and they are keen for him to return to work and he is considering a phased return to work. While previously a keen golfer, Joe has not managed to play a full round of golf as his stamina is still diminished. This has resulted in him continuing to employ his coping strategies regarding his negative thinking about whether he will be able to play golf again. Because of this intervention there have been changes at the person level. Joe is less fearful and more positive about his future and this has resulted in his family/community life being more normal with him engaging more in family roles. With the increase in his social contact at the golf club this reinforced his wider social and community participation.

References

Borrell-Carrio F, Suchman A, Epstein R M 2004 The biopsychosocial model 25 years later; principles, practice and scientific inquiry. Annals of Family Medicine 2(6):576–582

Christiansen C, Baum C 1997 Occupational therapy enabling function and well-being. Thorofare, New Jersey

Cook F M, Hassenkamp A 2000 Active rehabilitation for chronic low back pain: the patient's perspective. Physiotherapy 86:61–67

Engel G 1977 The need for a new medical model: a challenge for biomedicine. Science 196:129–136

Engel G 1980 The clinical application of the biopsychosocial model. American Journal of Psychiatry 137:535–544

Feaver S, Creek J 1993 Models of practice in occupational therapy. Part 2: what use are they? British Journal of Occupational Therapy 56(2):59–63

Hagedorn R 1997 Foundations for practice in occupational therapy, 2nd edn. Churchill Livingstone, Edinburgh

Kielhofner G 1995 A model of human occupation: theory and application, 2nd edn. Lippincott Williams and Wilkins, Baltimore

Kielhofner G 2002 A model of human occupation: theory and application, 3rd edn. Lippincott Williams and Wilkins, Baltimore

Kortman B 1995 The eye of the beholder models in occupational therapy model. British Journal of Occupational Therapy 58(12):532–536

McLaren N 1998 A critical view of the biopsychosocial model. Australian and New Zealand Journal of Psychiatry 32:86–72

Smith T W, Ruiz J M 2002 Psychosocial influences on the development and course of coronary disease: Current status and implications for research and practice. Journal of Consulting and Clinical Psychology 70:548–568

Suls J, Rothman A 2004 Evolution of the biopsychosocial model: prospects and challenges for health psychology. Health Psychology 23(2):119–125

Taylor R R 2005 Cognitive behavioural therapy for chronic illness and disability. Kluwer, New York

Waddell G 1987 A clinical model for the treatment of low back pain. Spine 12:632–643

White P 2005 Biopsychosocial medicine. Oxford University Press, Oxford

Biomedical links between cognitions and behaviour

Jan S Gill

3

Introduction

The barriers that historically rigidly delineated the separate territories of the neurophysiologist and the psychologist are being eroded allowing an appreciation of the multitude of physiological changes which occur within the substance of the brain, and which underpin the very essence of our mind's activity. Recent research findings, including those resulting from the use of non-invasive techniques such as brain-imaging technology, raise the possibility that the early years of the 21st century may herald real progress in our understanding of the pathological changes characterizing a range of psychiatric conditions. Hopefully a clearer and reasoned rationale for the most appropriate therapeutic approaches will emerge.

In order to more fully understand the link between thinking, emotion, behaviour and physiology, this chapter will consider research evidence relevant to the neurobiology of two conditions, anxiety and depression. This information will be preceded by a simplified view of pertinent aspects of brain physiology followed by a brief consideration of relevant functional neuroanatomy.

Aspects of brain physiology

We will begin by considering how brain activity is described from a physiological perspective. This view sees the brain as a mass of millions of body cells, i.e. nerve cells interacting and communicating with each other. Nerve cells, also known as neurones, are special for they can produce electrical signals which pass rapidly along a thin extension from the neurone called an axon. This axon can be likened to an electrical wire that reaches out towards neighbouring neurones. The axon does not actually touch the targeted neurone. Instead, the axon's electrical signal promotes the release of a chemical and it is this chemical, or more correctly neurotransmitter, which makes the final contact with the target neurone. The released neurotransmitter is able to bring about a change in the activity of the target neurone. In this way, electrically and then chemically, neurones communicate and influence each other.

What is the consequence of this neurone activity? Electrical and chemical communication between neurones in the various brain areas results in what we recognize as actions or thoughts. Every thought and action has a physical corollary in the brain. This is just as true for the muscular activity we associate with, say, physically smiling or the 'feel good factor' and mood that evoked our smile. In the clinical context this physiological perspective links malfunctions in the release of neurotransmitters and the consequent altered communication of neurones to pathology and psychiatric disturbance.

This model of brain activity also predicts that the manipulation of the levels of brain chemicals (the neurotransmitters referred to above) can so alter the interaction of the component neurones in the brain that a change in behaviour and (of relevance to this chapter) mood can be produced. Man, over the centuries by his designed and serendipitous use of chemicals (drugs), legal and illegal, has done exactly that.

Our next point of relevance to brain physiology relates to 'brain mapping'. Early brain research attempted to link neurones located within certain anatomical areas of the brain to specific human functions, e.g. neurones at the rear of the brain have been linked with the processing of visual information; those in the frontal regions of the brain with judgement, personality etc. Topographical maps of the brain surface were produced. However, it is now recognized that the true situation is much more complex and that these early maps, while useful, are nevertheless potentially misleading. The complex inward and outward manifestations we recognize as any aspect of human behaviour, e.g. mood, involve the interplay and communication of many brain areas. Thus a therapeutic approach which attempts to link mood to one single, identifiable area of the brain, where pathology will produce a particular mood disorder and which pharmaceuticals will discretely target to elicit a beneficial effect, is seriously misguided.

A final but very important aspect of neurone activity that we should consider is the phenomenon of plasticity. Plasticity relates to the ability of the brain connections to be 'reshaped' or moulded. The wiring of the brain, which we are viewing as the connections between neurones, is not 'set in stone' for the duration of life, but rather, is subject to reshaping. New wiring connections can be made and existing ones can be broken. In other words the functioning wiring patterns of the brain can be modified, fashioned by experience and by life itself. This is very evident in the developing child brain but, it should be stressed, is also evident in adults. The potential of the effective therapist to impact positively on this property of the brain cannot be overstressed. The well-documented recovery changes evident in the brain following stroke intervention therapy bear testament to this fact. Unfortunately the plasticity of the brain also makes it vulnerable; it may literally amass, and be influenced by, the scars of the emotional side of life, emphasizing the impact of the enduring nature of psychological distress on the brain.

We now proceed to a brief review of the structure of the brain and a summary of the functions linked with each brain region.

Relevant neuroanatomy

Regions of the brain associated with mood and emotion

Two large (cerebral) hemispheres dominate the view of the brain. The outermost layer of these hemispheres is referred to as the cerebral cortex (see Figure 3.1)

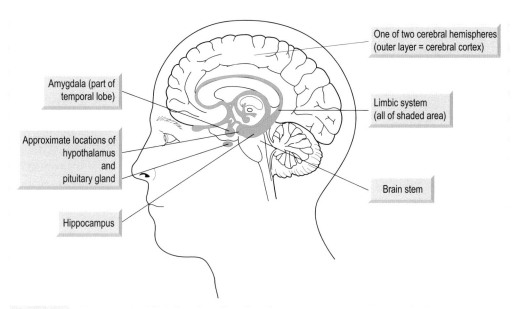

Figure 3.1 ● Diagrammatic view of the human brain (viewed from the side) to show limbic system (shaded area), cerebral cortex and brain stem.

and is linked to 'higher' functions and sophisticated processing of information. But, lying inside the hemispheres, around the core of the front region of the brain is an inner circuit of interconnected structures called the limbic system (the shaded area in Figure 3.1). The limbic system has long been linked to our emotions and their expression.

The limbic system can be viewed as connecting above, to regions of higher function in the cerebral cortex, and communicating below to the hypothalamus (with links to the body's endocrine system) and brain stem (with links to the nerves leading to the body). Armed with this brief summary of its anatomical position one can appreciate that the emotions originating within the limbic system can coordinate a massive body-wide response involving hormones and nerve activity (see Case Study 2.2 in Chapter 2). The many physical signs of emotion we recognize in our bodies result in blushing, racing heart, sweating etc.

We can illustrate these limbic-system-orchestrated effects by considering the body's response to a stressful event. This might be the sight of something threatening, a wild animal, or the recall of a very traumatic memory. Stress, from whatever source, is processed within the brain and evokes responses summarized as the 'fright, fight, flight' response. The need of an animal to survive is paramount and the neurone signals pass down through the hypothalamus within the limbic system to the pituitary gland. This endocrine gland, attached to the base of the brain, is in turn responsible for the ensuing secretion, directly and indirectly, of many body hormones. (This is often referred to as the hypothalamic pituitary axis, or HPA.) The action of these hormones is to induce body metabolic changes to support the individual's response to stress, e.g. the running away from the animal.

Simultaneously, links from the limbic system down to the brain stem initiate activity in our nervous system. This can result in activation of our muscles (to allow rapid movement away from the wild animal) but also nervous activity of the internal parts of the body again to support our response, metabolically and physically. This nervous response affects virtually every body tissue. The changes are reinforced by the outpouring of adrenaline from the adrenal gland.

In summary, a relatively quick, survival-orientated, widespread response coordinated by the limbic system and manifest by both the nervous and endocrine systems, is activated in the body. However, it must be emphasized that this response can occur when there is no clear external stressor; it can also occur when there is 'no place to run'. In both situations the bodily response still occurs as before but its effect potentially changes from being survival orientated and desirable to counter-productive and damaging, potentially leading to physical and psychological problems.

One component of the hormonal response described above is of particular relevance to our later discussion. It is corticotropin-releasing hormone (CRH). CRH is released from the hypothalamus and in turn, stimulates the release of the hormone adrenocorticotropic hormone (ACTH) from the anterior pituitary gland. This hormone travels in the blood to act on the adrenal cortex (a gland on the kidney) so releasing the major stress hormone cortisol into blood. Cortisol, the final product in this complex sequence of endocrine gland activity, acts within the body to promote many of the metabolic changes supporting our 'fright, fight, flight' reaction referred to above. However, actions of CRH, additional to that leading to cortisol production are recognized. CRH may act elsewhere in the brain and this action of CRH has been directly linked to the pathology of both depression and anxiety. We shall refer to CRH again in later sections.

It must be emphasized that the above description inevitably describes a 'top down' response from the limbic system. However, feedback to this emotional centre from the body through nerves and blood-borne chemicals is also vital. Additionally, the higher centres within the cerebral cortex influence, and are influenced by, the limbic system. In simplistic terms the intensity of our stress response may be modified positively or negatively by cognitive processing and by the feedback to the brain of body hormones etc. Intuitively this point seems correct. Our cognitive ability to dismiss the approaching 'wild animal' as a picture, or as a soft toy may restrain our stress response.

A simplistic model of limbic connections with complex interacting circuits of activity is presented in Figure 3.2.

Evidence from studies shows that directly stimulating parts of the limbic system results in vocalization in animals; in man this is linked to actual emotional experiences, e.g. to the emotional experience of pain, feelings of fear, panic and a sense of foreboding (Price et al 1996). Positron emission tomography studies (PET) have demonstrated that anger-inducing events (Dougherty et al 1999) or listening to discordant music (Blood et al 1999) have been linked to activity in the limbic system.

The particular roles of two components of the limbic system merit further description.

The amygdala (see Figure 3.1) has a pivotal role in organizing the stress behavioural responses which are manifest through the nervous and hormonal responses to sensory threat and outlined above. Through links from the amygdala to brain regions involved in muscle control, movements of an instinctive nature such as defence or attack stances can be initiated. The nervous signal carrying 'details 'of the sensory threat (stressor), appears to reach the amygdala by two routes; the first,

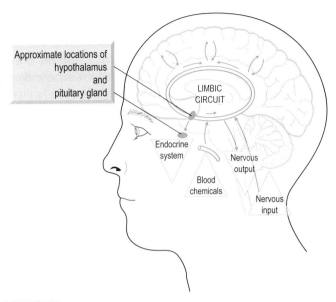

Figure 3.2 Schematic representation of some of the interconnections between the limbic system and other parts of the nervous system.

direct route, supplies unprocessed, sensory information and the amygdala appears to organize a rapid, essentially protective response. In man this reaction to visual and auditory sensory input may explain our subconscious fear response (Ledoux et al 1989). Animal survival is favoured by this rapid, effective fear response and Ninian et al (2002) describe it as' emotional and non-cognitive (automatic, predetermined and species typical)' (p 69). In man visual and auditory sensory input are particularly important, in lower animals olfactory information is crucial.

The second source of sensory information arrives at the amygdala after initial processing by higher cortical sensory centres. It is, in relative terms, delayed having undergone more sophisticated processing by the higher cortical regions to ensure a more reasoned response.

Within the amygdala the processing of the sensory information will be influenced by memories, body state etc. In addition, virtually permanent traces for fear conditioning are established (Maren 1999). Studies implicate a role for the amygdala in:

* the recall of emotional memories (Canli et al 2000)
* the actual emotional experience (Gloor et al 1982)
* aggressive behaviour
* our unconscious ability to interpret fearful facial expression.

All of the above implicate a role for the amygdala in the process of aversive emotional learning (Adolphs et al 1999). It is not surprising that damage to the amygdala is associated with 'flattened emotions' (Bechara et al 1995).

The second structure worthy of note is the hippocampus (see Figure 3.1), a structure with extensive links to the cerebral cortex and the amygdala. It is thought to

If the proposal that anxiety can be described as an overactive stress response is correct, then we can speculate that the source of the problem may arise at more then one level. It may result from (i) the failure of the higher cortical circuits to cognitively 'restrain' the amygdala, (ii) dominating amygdala-orchestrated behaviour or (iii) overactive brain stem links to the mechanisms organizing the body response to stress. In the case of the picture of a wild animal initiating the stress response, the knowledge that it is just a picture may be insufficient to prevent the amygdala-orchestrated response. Similarly, simple awareness that your body is breathing rapidly or that your heart is racing, may in itself be stress-inducing.

Thus in summary, while the model depicting anxiety as a condition resulting from an overactive stress response is attractive, it is important to emphasize that the system does not work exclusively 'top down'. The trigger for anxiety can come from a variety of sources. Thus overactive brain-stem 'panic' responses may well impact on our ability to cognitively process incoming sensory information. Ninian et al (2002) have discussed sensory somatic triggers ('bottom up') and cognitive ('top down') influences and highlight that evidence suggests that the sensitivity of the amygdala can in a sense be 'set' by cognitive mechanisms. There is also good evidence for changes being induced in this control of our stress response by life itself. Early experiences may contribute to the establishment of a 'set point' for the stress response which critically determines the magnitude of our stress response as an adult (reviewed by Charney 2003). This may explain the individual variation in response to stress and the possibility of changing vulnerability through cognitive mechanisms.

As we have noted, the neural and endocrine signals that are produced in response to amygdala input are initiated from the brain stem. Within this area there is a collection of neurones with a major stimulatory influence on this panic response: the locus coeruleus. Many neurones within this structure employ the neurotransmitter noradrenaline. Thus the rationale for the early anxiolytic (anxiety-reducing) drugs is clear; drugs which decrease the activity of the neurotransmitter noradrenaline decrease the influence of the locus coeruleus and should be anxiolytic.

The role of the hippocampus in our model of anxiety merits further discussion. As noted, it is found within the limbic system and makes several connections with the amygdala. Along with several other brain areas, the hippocampus may endow us with the ability to judge the significance of a threat based on our past experience, and if it is unusual, the need for higher processing. Critically, the hippocampus may exert a modulatory role on the endocrine stress response for it contains receptors sensitive to the stress hormone cortisol. In response to increased blood levels of the stress hormone cortisol, the hippocampus can, via connections to the hypothalamus, effectively switch off secretion of CRH and thereby cortisol production. In other words it may 'tone down' the stress response.

If the hippocampus were damaged we might lose this restraining action and this could impact on our ability to avoid over-reaction; we would fail to put a stressor in context. Significantly, there is evidence of damage to the hippocampus being reported in studies where animals have been subjected to sustained stress (Sapolsky 1996). Several studies involving human subjects have reported reductions in the volume of hippocampal tissue in post-traumatic stress disorder (PTSD) following military action (Bremner et al 1995, Gurvits et al 1996), childhood abuse (Bremner et al 1997b, Stein et al 1997) or childhood sexual abuse (Bremner et al 2003).

The underlying pathology may not be an overactive HPA, rather, one that is unrestrained. Evidence consistent with an overactive stress response being present is the report of elevated levels of CRH in the fluid surrounding the brain (cerebrospinal fluid) in long-term PTSD (Bremner et al 1997a; Baker et al 1999).

Another study has implicated the hippocampus in the pathology of social phobia or social anxiety disorder. Poor communication between the hippocampus and the amygdala leading to faulty contextualization of fear may be relevant (Gray & McNaughton 1996).

This model for the pathophysiology of stress may also be employed to explain the rationale for the anxiolytic properties of drugs like the benzodiazepines (BDZ). Some of the neurones which restrain this brain stress pathway release the neurotransmitter gamma amino butyric acid (GABA) (see Figure 3.3). The action of this neurotransmitter is to inhibit the release of CRH from neurones within the hypothalamus. In turn the stress response is diminished (Calogero et al 1988). By this reasoning, drugs that enhance the activity of GABA are associated with anxiolytic actions, those which inhibit or prevent it, with anxiogenic properties. The BDZ drugs act to improve the response within the brain to any released GABA, the release of CRH is reduced, the stress pathway is less active and an anxiolytic effect achieved.

Panic attacks have also been linked from a pathological perspective to overactivation of the HPA. Some evidence is emerging to link changes in GABA sensitivity to panic disorder (Davis et al 1997, Malizia et al 1998).

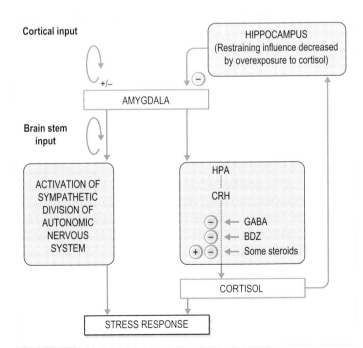

Figure 3.3 Diagrammatic view of the interaction of factors within the brain which may lead to the overactivation of the stress pathway and thereby the expression of anxiety symptoms (GABA = gamma amino butyric acid, HPA = hypothalamic axis, BDZ = benzodiazepine drugs, CRH = corticotropin-releasing hormone).

The proposal is that in depression the axis is again overactive. One supporting argument is that many of the symptoms which characterize stress, e.g. changes in appetite, decreased interest in sex, alertness being replaced by anxiety etc. also characterize depression. The implication is that levels of a controlling factor in the axis (CRH), and/or the product of the axis, cortisol, are raised and it is their actions elsewhere in the brain that cause depression. In support of this proposal is the finding that in response to CRH infusion there is evidence of increased arousal, reduced appetite and sleep disturbances, symptoms common in depression (Arborelius et al 1999, Holsboer 2001). Linking this with the knowledge that compounds that block the action of CRH may have antidepressant actions (Wong et al 2000) appears to lead to the idea that hyperactivity of the HPA may also be relevant to depression pathophysiology.

Barden (2004) suggests that antidepressant drugs act not in the way outlined by the monoamine hypothesis, but by ensuring that the hormonal axis producing cortisol is more sensitive to the restraining action of feedback. The extent to which this theory may underlie all depression subtypes is questionable. Opinions vary. Excessive activation of the cortisol hormonal axis is reported to characterize only 50% of cases of depression (Nestler et al 2002), while two studies have reported that it is more common in bipolar than unipolar depression (Rybakowski & Twardowska 1999, Rush et al 1996). Others have linked depression to an abnormal diurnal rhythm of cortisol secretion (Cervantes et al 2001) or high levels in the morning (Harris et al 2000), while Schatzberg (2004) reported that the relaxation of the axis from 1 pm to 4 pm – usually evident in non-depressed subjects, was often not found with psychotic depressed subjects.

In considering the impact of an assumed overactive hormonal axis it is necessary to restress the important links this axis has with the hippocampus. Cortisol binds to cells within the hypothalamus and pituitary and the hippocampus, to regulate by negative feedback, its own production. High levels of cortisol effectively alert the hippocampus to initiate its restraining action on the HPA and so reduce cortisol production. An 'over the top' stress response is avoided. However, unrelenting high cortisol levels as in chronic stress may cause tissue damage in the hippocampus (McEwen 2000, Sapolsky 2000). It is less able to exert the level of inhibitory control and depression is promoted.

In terms of the behavioural response to overactivity of the HPA, it could be that either or both of CRH and cortisol act in other areas of the brain to cause the recognizable symptoms of depression. CRH antagonists have been investigated as potential antidepressants in humans (Zobel et al 2000) and in rats (Holsboer 2001, 2003).

Neuronal atrophy and cell death hypothesis

This third hypothesis to explain the pathophysiology of depression has recently gained prominence. The focus here is not on transmitter system anomalies per se but instead on the processes within all neurons that are vital to their survival and development. We have already mentioned the topic of plasticity. This is the reshaping of the brain that occurs during development and learning etc. In practice it means that some neurones are identified as important, their connections (axons etc.) are strengthened and established. Other neurones may be seen as surplus to requirements and as brain pathways become established these healthy, but not required, neurones will be allowed to die. This is the orderly process of 'natural' or programmed cell death (apoptosis).

The neuronal atrophy and cell-death hypothesis of depression was proposed by Duman et al (2001). In many ways this model appears to neatly link many aspects of the present understanding of the neurobiology of depression. In essence it proposes that the effects of stress (high levels of CRH and cortisol), genetic influences etc., shift the balance of chemical signals within neurones from development and 'moulding', i.e. survival, to 'suicide' or apoptosis, i.e. neurone loss. The consequence is the appearance of symptoms reflecting the lost role of the missing neurons – in other words loss of neurones in areas of the brain important to mood and motivation lead to the classic symptoms of depression.

There is indeed some evidence for an effect of stress or cortisol on the numbers of cells in regions of the brain we have already discussed as playing an important role in the stress response. Cortisol may prejudice the processes of neurone birth and growth, vital to hippocampal function and, in addition, to encourage cell death (Gould et al 2000). Animal studies provide evidence of stress-induced changes in hippocampal tissue which appear to be reversed by antidepressant medication (Kuroda and McEwen 1998, Norrholm & Oulmet 2001). In frontal cortical tissue Glitz et al (2002) suggest links between the effects of chronic stress, tissue damage and the impairment of working memory evident in depression.

One important positive influence on cell viability is brain-derived neurotrophic factor (BDNF). This molecule, present within neurones, prevents, by a complex series of intracellular reactions, apoptosis. It thus has a vital role to play in cell survival. Activation of the stress pathway may lead to a fall in the levels of BDNF and apoptosis is favoured (Manji et al 2001). In this theory long-term use of antidepressant drugs is effective not by raising neurotransmitter levels in critical areas of the brain but instead by promoting BDNF production so favouring cell survival. The antidepressant lithium is proposed to promote changes which prevent the death of vital neurones. Long-term use of a range of antidepressants is assumed to promote BDNF production.

Another molecule found in neurones (c-AMP response element binding protein, CREB) is also known to promote the production of BDNF. Increased levels of CREB in the neurones of the hippocampus and other brain areas have been attributed to the action of certain antidepressants (Nibuya et al 1996, Thome et al 2000). Electroconvulsive therapy has also been linked to beneficial effects on CREB production (Nibuya et al 1995, 1996). These findings may explain why the pharmacological action of some antidepressant drugs on neurotransmitter levels is often evident relatively quickly but the hope for remission of depressant symptoms may take several weeks to act. The real therapeutic benefit has resulted from drug-induced but time-consuming changes in cell chemistry.

A diagrammatic view of factors which may be relevant to the aetiology of depression is shown in Figure 3.4.

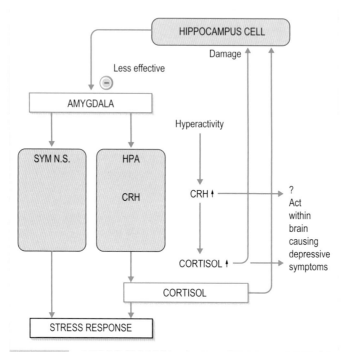

Figure 3.4 Diagrammatic view of the interaction of factors within the brain stress response which may lead to overactivation of the body's stress response and thereby the expression of depressive symptoms (SYM N.S. = sympathetic nervous system, HPA = hypothalamic pituitary axis, CRH = corticotropin-releasing hormone).

Conclusions

Clear overlap in the underlying pathology of the two conditions of depression and anxiety is beginning to emerge as our investigation progresses. Our knowledge has been enhanced by evidence produced by human brain imaging techniques. We can be hopeful of novel, more specific and effective therapies in anxieties and depression. It is likely that factors such as gender and genetic profiles may be two of several crucial factors that explain whether or not the pathology caused by an excessive stress response is revealed as depressive and/or anxiety symptoms. While this book's emphasis is on the application of CBT to physiotherapy and occupational therapy practice, our understanding of the neurophysiology of anxiety and depression will give a fuller understanding of the interplay between biological, psychological and social systems as described by the biopsychosocial model.

References

Adolphs R, Tranel D, Hamann S et al 1999 Recognition of facial emotion in nine individu- als with bilateral amygdala damage. Neuropsy- chologia 37:1111–1117

Arborelius L, Owens M J, Plotsky P M et al 1999 The role of corticotropin-releasing factor in depression and anxiety disorders. Journal of Endocrinology 160:1–12

Baker D G, West S A, Nicholson W E et al 1999 Serial CSF corticotropin-releasing hormone levels and adrenocortical activity in combat veterans with post-traumatic stress disorder. American Journal of Psychiatry 156:585–588

Barden N 2004 Implications of the hypothalamic-pituitary-adrenal axis in the pathophysiology of depression. Journal of Psychiatry and Neuroscience 29(3):185–193

Bardo M T 1998 Neuropharmacological mechanisms of drug reward: beyond dopamine in the nucleus accumbens. Critical Review of Neurobiology 12:37–67

Bechara A, Tranel D, Damasio H et al 1995 Double dissociation of conditioning and declarative knowledge relative to the amygdala and hippocampus in humans. Science 269:1115–1118

Blood A J, Zatorre R J, Bermudez P et al 1999 Emotional responses to pleasant and unpleasant music correlate with activity in paralimbic brain regions. Nature Neuroscience 2:382–387

Bremner J D, Randall P, Scott T M et al 1995 MRI-based measurement hippocampal volume patients with combat-related post traumatic stress disorder. American Journal of Psychiatry 152:973–981

Bremner J D, Licinio J, Darnell A et al 1997a Elevated CSF corticotrophin-releasing factor concentrations in post-traumatic stress disorder. American Journal of Psychiatry 154:624–629

Bremner J D, Randall P, Vermetten E et al 1997b Magnetic resonance imaging-based measurement of hippocampal volume in post traumatic stress disorder related to childhood physical and sexual abuse – a preliminary report. Biological Psychiatry 41:23–32

Bremner J D, Vythilingam M, Vermetten E et al 2003 MRI and PET study of deficits in hippocampal structure and function in women with childhood sexual abuse and posttraumatic stress disorder. American Journal of Psychiatry 160:924–932

Calogero A E, Gallucci W T, Chousos G P et al 1988 Interaction between GABAergic neurotransmission and rat hypothalamic corticotrophin releasing hormone secretion in vitro. Brain Research 463:28–36

Canli T, Zhao Z, Brewer J et al 2000 Event-related activation in the human amygdala associates with later memory for individual emotional experience. Journal of Neuroscience 20:RC99

Cardno A G, Marshall E J, Coid B et al 1999 Heritability estimates for psychotic disorders. The Maudsley twin psychosis series. Archives of General Psychiatry 56:162–168

Cervantes P, Gelber S, Kin F N et al 2001 Circadian secretion of cortisol in bipolar disorder. Journal of Psychiatry Neuroscience 26:411–416

Charney D S 2003 Neuroanatomical circuits modulating fear and anxiety behaviours. Acta Psychiatrica Scandinavica 108(suppl 417):38–50

Coppen A 1967 The biochemistry of affective disorders. British Journal of Psychiatry 113(504):1237–1264

Davis M, Walker D L, Lee Y 1997 Roles of the amygdala and bed nucleus of the stria terminalis in fear and anxiety measured with the acoustic startle reflex. Annals of the New York Academy of Science 831:305–315

Dougherty D D, Shin L M, Alpert N M et al 1999 Anger in healthy men: a PET study using script-driven imagery. Biological Psychiatry 46:466–472

Duman R S, Malberg J, Nakagawa S 2001 Regulation of adult neurogenesis by psychotropic drugs and stress. Journal of Pharmacology and Experimental Therapy 299:401–407

Fava M, Kendler K S 2000 Major depressive disorder. Neuron 28:335–341

Glitz D A, Manji H K, Moore G J 2002 Mood disorders: treatment-induced changes in brain neurochemistry and structure. Seminars in Clinical Neuropsychiatry 7:269–280

Gloor P, Olivier A, Quesney L F et al 1982 The role of the limbic system in experiential phenomena of temporal lobe epilepsy. Annals of Neurology 12:129–144

Gould E, Tanapat P, Rydel T et al 2000 Regulation of hippocampal neurogenesis in adulthood. Biological Psychiatry 48:715–720

Gray J A, McNaughton N 1996 The neuropsychology of anxiety: reprise. Nebraska Symposium on Motivation 43:61–134

Gumnick J F, Nemeroff C B 2000 Problems with currently available antidepressants. Journal of Clinical Psychiatry 61(Suppl 10):5–15

Gutman S A, Haynes J L 2002 Unipolar depression: a literature review of the most current epidemiological theories. Occupational Therapy in Mental Health 18(2):45–79

Gurvits T V, Shenton M E, Hokama H et al 1996 Magnetic resonance imaging study of hippocampal volume in chronic combat-related post traumatic stress disorder. Biological Psychiatry 40:1091–1099

Harris T O, Borsanyi S, Messari S et al 2000 Morning cortisol as a risk factor for subsequent major depressive disorder in adult women. British Journal of Psychiatry 177:505–510

Holsboer F 2001 Stress, hypercortisolism and corticosteroid receptors in depression: implications for therapy. Journal of Affective Disorders 62:77–91

Holsboer F 2003 High-quality antidepressant discovery by understanding stress hormone physiology. Annals of the New York Academy of Sciences 1007:394–404

Kendler K S, Pedersen N L, Neale M C et al 1995 A pilot Swedish twin study of affective illness including hospital and population-ascertained subsamples: results of model fitting. Behavior Genetics 25:217–232

Koob G F, Heinrichs S C 1999 A role for corticotropin releasing factor and urocortin in behavioural responses to stressors. Brain Research 848:141–152

Kuroda Y, McEwen B S 1998 Effect of chronic restraint stress and tianoptine on growth factors, growth-associated protein-43 and microtubule-associated protein 2 mRNA expression in rat hippocampus. Molecular Brain Research 59:35–39

Ledoux J E, Romanski L, Xagoraris A 1989 Indelibility of subcortical emotional memories. Journal of Cognitive Neurosciences 1:238–243

Lesch K P 2004 Gene-environment interaction and the genetics of depression. Journal of Psychiatry and Neuroscience 29(3):174–184

McEwan B S 2000 Allostasis and allostatic load: implications for neuropsychopharmacology. Neuropsychopharmacology 22:108–124

Malizia A L, Cunningham V J, Bell C J et al 1998 Decreased brain GABA-benzodiazepine receptor binding in panic disorder. Archives of General Psychiatry 55:715–720

Manji HK, Drevets WC, Charney DS 2001 The cellular neurobiology of depression. Nature Medicine 7:541–547

Maren S 1999 Long-term potentiation in the amygdala: a mechanism for emotional learning and memory. Trends in Neuroscience 22:561–567

Naranjo C A, Tremblay L K, Busto U E 2001 The role of the brain reward system in depression. Progress in Neuropsychopharmacology and Biological Psychiatry 25(4):781–823

Nemeroff C B 2002 Recent advances in the neurobiology of depression. Psychopharmacology Bulletin 36(suppl 2):6–23

Nestler E J, Barrot M, DiLeone R J et al 2002 Neurobiology of depression. Neuron 34:13–25

Nibuya M, Morfnobu S, Durman R S 1995 Regulation of BDNF and trkB mRNA in rat brain by chronic electroconvulsive seizure and antidepressant drug treatments. Journal of Neuroscience 15:7539–7547

Nibuya M, Nestler E J, Duman R S 1996 Chronic antidepressant administration increases the expression of cAMP response element binding protein (CREB) in rat hippocampus. Journal of Neuroscience 16:2365–2372

Ninian P T, Feigon S A, Knight B 2002 Neurobiology and mechanisms of antidepressant treatment response in anxiety. Psychopharmacology Bulletin 36(suppl 3):67–78

Norrholm S D, Oulmet C C 2001 Altered dendritic spine density in animal models of depression and in response to antidepressant treatment. Synapse 42:151–163

Parker G B, Brotchie H L 2004 From diathesis to dimorphism: the biology of gender differences in depression. The Journal of Nervous and Mental Disease 192(3): 210–216

Price J L, Carmichael S T, Drevets W C 1996 Networks related to the orbital and medial prefrontal cortex: a substrate for emotional behaviour? Progress in Brain Research 197:523–536

Rush A J, Giles D E, Schlesser M A et al 1996 The dexamethasone suppression test in patients with mood disorders. Journal of Clinical Psychiatry 57:470–484

Rybakowski J K, Twardowska K 1999 The dexamethasone/corticotropin-releasing hormone test in depression in bipolar and unipolar affective illness. Journal of Psychiatric Research 33:363–370

Sanders A R, Detera-Wadleigh S D, Gershon E S 1999 Molecular genetics of mood disorders. In: Charney D S, Nestler E J, Bunney B S (eds) Neurobiology of Mental Illness. Oxford University Press, New York, pp 299–316

Sandford J J, Argyropoulos S V, Nutt D J 2000 The psychobiology of anxiolytic drugs. Part 1: basic neurobiology. Pharmacology and Therapeutics 88:197–212

Sapolsky R M 1996 Why stress is bad for your brain. Science 273:749–750

Sapolsky R M 2000 Glucocorticoids and hippocampal atrophy in neuropsychiatric disorders. Archives of General Psychiatry 57:925–935

Schatzberg A 2004 An update on glucocorticoid antagonist in depression: research in depression and mood disorders, Program and abstracts of the international Congress of Biological Psychiatry Sydney Australia Symposium 24

Schildkraut J F, Gordon E K, Durell J 1965 Catecholamine metabolism in affective disorders: I. Normetanephrine and VMA excretion in depressed patients treated with imipramine. Journal of Psychiatric Research 3:213–228

Schulkin J, Gold P W, McEwen B S 1998 Induction of corticotrophin-releasing hormone gene expression by glucocorticoids: implication for understanding the states of fear and anxiety and allostatic load. Psychoneuroendocrinology 23:219–243

Stein M B, Koverola C, Hanna C et al 1997 Hippocampal volume in women victimized by childhood sexual abuse. Psychological Medicine 27:951–959

Tekin S, Cummings J L 2002 Frontal-subcortical neuronal circuits and clinical neuropsychiatry: An update. Journal of Psychosomatic Research 53:647–654

Thome J, Sakai N, Shin K, et al 2000 cAMP response element-mediated gene transcription is upregulated by chronic antidepressant treatment. Journal of Neuroscience 20:4030–4036

Winkler D, Pjrek E, Heiden A et al 2004 Gender differences in the psychopathology of depressed inpatients. European Archives of Psychiatry and Clinical Neuroscience 254(4):209–214

Wong, M L, Kling M A, Munson P J et al 2000 Pronounced and sustained central hypernoradrenergic function in major depression with melancholic features: relation to hypercortisolism and corticotropin releasing hormone. Proceedings of the National Academy of Sciences USA 97:325–330

Woodward J, Chang J Y, Janak P et al 1999 Mesolimbic neuronal activity across behavioral states. Annals of the New York Academy of Sciences 877:91–112

Zadina J E, Martin-Schild S, Gerall A A et al 1999 Endomorphins: novel endogenous μ-opiate receptor agonists in regions of high μ-opiate receptor density. Annals of the New York Academy of Science 877:136–144

Zobel A W, Nickel T, Kunzel H E et al 2000 Effects of the high-affinity corticotropin-releasing hormone receptor 1 antagonist R121919 in major depression. The first 20 patients treated. Journal of Psychiatric Research 34:171–181

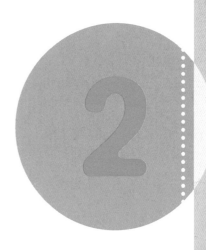

Part 2

Practical application

51

Cognitive–behavioural therapy for depression

4

Kate Davidson and Anne Joice

Prevalence

Depression is one of the most commonly occurring mental health problems and is recognized as a leading cause of disability throughout the world (Murray & Lopez 1996). There may be up to 5% of the population suffering from depression at any one time. Women have a much greater lifetime risk for depression, 1.7 to 2.7 greater than men, with an increased risk of first onset of depression from early adolescence up to the age of mid fifties (Burt & Stein 2002).

What is depression?

Depression is a normal mood state, familiar to most people. Depression can range from minor mood disturbance – a low mood accompanied with negative thoughts – to more severe depression where an individual will experience more symptoms and problems. If an individual experiences five or more symptoms over a two-week period, a formal diagnosis of depression is given. Box 4.1 lists the diagnostic features of major depression. A minority of patients referred to waiting-list control groups in a clinical trial of interventions are known to improve spontaneously over two months and this number rises to around half of all patients in these studies within six months (Posternak & Miller 2001). Although around half of people with depression therefore recover from depression in less than three months, a substantial minority will experience a more chronic course of illness with 22% remaining depressed two years later (Keller et al 1984). Depression is now known to be a condition that reoccurs (Solomon et al 2000). Roughly half of those affected by depression will have no further episodes but the corollary is that at least 50% of people following their first episode of major depression will go on to have at least one more episode (Kupfer 1991). After a second episode the risk of further relapse rises to 70% and to 90% if there is a third episode (Kupfer 1991). If depression begins at or before the age of twenty, individuals are thought to have increased vulnerability to relapse (Giles et al 1989). This suggests that many patients with depression will have a relapsing course and may suffer over many years (Akiskal 1986).

Box 4.1

Diagnostic criteria for Major Depressive Disorder

(adapted from DSM-IV, American Psychiatric Association 1994)

Five (or more) of the following symptoms have been present during the same two-week period and represent a change from previous functioning. The following symptoms should be present most of the day or nearly every day and result in significant distress or impairment of functioning. The symptoms are not due to bereavement or due to the direct physiological effects of a substance. At least one of the symptoms is either (1) depressed mood or (2) loss of interest or pleasure.

- Depressed mood most of the day
- Markedly diminished interest or pleasure in all, or almost all, activities
- Significant weight loss when not dieting or weight gain
- Insomnia or hypersomnia
- Psychomotor retardation or agitation
- Fatigue or loss of energy
- Feelings of worthlessness or excessive or inappropriate guilt
- Diminished ability to think or concentrate, or indecisiveness
- Recurrent thoughts of death, recurrent suicidal ideation without a specific plan, or a suicide attempt or plan for committing suicide.

Depression is evident in primary-care settings and in a large variety of health-care settings apart from mental health services. For example, around 15% of adult medical inpatients met ICD-9 criteria for major depressive disorder (Feldman et al 1987). Around 8 to 10% of patient consultations in primary care (Blacker & Clare 1987) are related to depression. This might suggest that patients themselves may not recognize that they are depressed or regard depressive symptoms, such as low mood, as being a normal accompaniment to physical problems. There is also evidence that people with depression would be embarrassed to consult their general practitioner and that individuals in the general population are ill-informed about the effectiveness of treatment (Priest et al 1996). Although there are efforts to reduce stigma associated with mental illness (Paykel et al 1998; Crisp 2000), ignorance and stigmatization of depression still exist, particularly towards older adults with mental illness (Davidson & Connery 2003).

By far the majority of people suffering from depression will receive treatment from their general practitioners. The most common form of treatment is antidepressant medication. This form of treatment is relatively inexpensive and relatively effective (see Chapter 3 for a fuller discussion). However, some patients do not want to take medication or cannot tolerate the side-effects of antidepressant medication. There are also some who would prefer to overcome depression through a talking therapy such as cognitive therapy, either with or without taking antidepressant medication.

The efficacy of cognitive–behavioural therapy for major depression

The best evidence of the effectiveness of cognitive–behavioural therapy comes from randomized controlled trials. Early studies of cognitive therapy demonstrated that cognitive therapy either on its own, or in combination with medication, was as effective as antidepressant medication (Blackburn et al 1986, Beck et al 1979) or more effective than antidepressant medication (Rush et al 1977, McLean & Hakstian 1979). Later studies also found that cognitive therapy was at least equivalent in efficacy to antidepressant medication (Hollon et al 1992) and antidepressant medication delivered by specialist or general practitioners or social work counselling (Scott & Freeman 1992). There is some evidence from early studies of psychological treatment of followed-up patients that a course of either cognitive therapy (Blackburn et al 1986) or interpersonal therapy may reduce the risk of future relapse (Elkin et al 1989, Evans et al 1992).

The NIMH Treatment of Depression Collaborative Research Program

One of the largest, and possibly most controversial of studies to be undertaken in depression was the National Institute of Mental Health's (NIMH) Treatment of Depression Collaborative Research Program (TDCRP). In this North American study, 239 unipolar depressed outpatients at three different sites were randomly allocated to one of four treatments. The treatment conditions were cognitive–behavioural therapy (CBT), imipramine plus clinical management (ICM), interpersonal psychotherapy (IPT) and a pill placebo control. The initial findings were that there were few differences at the end of treatment among the four conditions (Elkin et al 1989). However, when severity of depression at the beginning of treatment was taken into account, those patients who received IPT and ICM had a better response than did patients who had received the pill placebo. CBT did not produce significantly greater benefit to more severely depressed patients. ICM was significantly superior to CBT for the more severely ill patients and IPT was also superior to CBT for the more severely depressed, but not functionally impaired patients (Elkin et al 1995). In addition, ICM was also superior to IPT for the more severely ill patients when using the severity criterion based on the Global Assessment Scale (GAS), though the special benefits of ICM did not extend beyond the treatment period.

The NIMH study has resulted in a debate about preferred treatment models, with advocates of drug therapy highlighting the superiority of the active drug treatment compared to pill placebo and CBT. With equal vociferousness, those who have an interest in psychotherapy argued that IPT, rather than CBT, is the treatment of choice in severe depression or that the differences between the conditions that were found were not robust. Reanalysis of the data further added to this debate. Klein & Ross (1993) and Elkin and her colleagues (1995) both re-examined the data using different types of analyses and both separately concluded that psychotherapy was inferior to drug treatment among the more severely depressed patients. However, to complicate matters further, Elkin et al (1989) had found that the more severely depressed patients at one of the three sites did very well with CBT and had similar scores to those receiving ICM, and that IPT had also had a very good effect at another site, suggesting that there may have been differences according to site for the effectiveness of the psychotherapy conditions. This raised the possibility of either allegiance to a brand of therapy and/or competence with which the psychological treatments were delivered in the study were important factors influencing clinical outcomes.

At follow-up of 18 months, there were no differences between any of the treatments in long-term outcome, regardless of initial severity of depression (Shea et al 1992). Long-term outcome was not particularly good for any of the treatment conditions in terms of those who completed treatment, had recovered and remained recovered (CBT 30%; IPT 26%; pill placebo 20%; ICM 19%). This indicates that CBT was as good as any of the other treatments in the longer term, though the results are not particularly striking in terms of overall clinical effectiveness. In addition, of those who received pharmacotherapy, over 30% dropped out of treatment and of those who remained in treatment, the majority did not recover. For those who did recover, 50% relapsed when medication was withdrawn (Jacobson & Hollon 1996).

Can CBT reduce relapse rates?

Several studies have suggested that cognitive therapy may reduce relapse rates in depression. A two-year follow-up of patients (Evans et al 1992) evaluated the impact of continuing medication in 107 unipolar depressed patients. In the acute phase of illness, patients had received either CBT alone, imipramine hydrochloride alone or combined treatment (Hollon et al 1992). At the end of the treatment all active conditions were equally effective and importantly, unlike the NIMH study cited above, no differences were detected in terms of symptomatic response, even in severely depressed patients, on patient-rated and clinician-rated measures. Patients treated with three months of CBT, either alone or in combination, had less than half the relapse rate of patients who had received three months of medication. The relapse rate after three months of CBT did not differ from that of patients provided with 15 months of medication.

Similar findings were demonstrated by Blackburn & Moore (1997) who treated 75 patients in three crossovers of treatment conditions. One group of patients received antidepressant medication in the acute phase followed by either antidepressants or CBT, or by CBT in the acute phase followed by CBT. In the acute phase, there were no differences in response to CBT or antidepressant medication and all groups showed significant improvement in symptoms. During the follow-up phase, there were also no differences in relapse rates between the group and all showed improvement with time, whether CBT followed acute treatment with CBT or not. So, rather than supporting the argument for long-term drug treatment, these studies support treating depression with CBT.

It is not uncommon for patients treated for depression with antidepressant medication to make only a partial response to treatment and to suffer high rates of relapse. Paykel and his colleagues (Paykel et al 1998) treated 158 patients with a recent episode of major depression who had partial remission of symptoms with antidepressant treatment but who had residual symptoms lasting between two and 18 months. Patients were randomized to one of two conditions, either clinical management alone or clinical management plus CBT. CBT reduced relapse rates for acute depression and persistent severe residual symptoms. At 68 weeks, only 29% of those who had received CBT had relapsed compared to 47% in the clinical management group, indicating that CBT benefits this group of patients who have traditionally been regarded as being difficult to treat because of their partial response to antidepressant medication. Although the additional CBT was more costly, it was more effective than clinical management (Scott et al 2003).

Summary

Case Study 4.1 demonstrates how effectively CBT can enhance the role of occupational therapy, or indeed physiotherapy in treating depression.

CASE STUDY 4.1

Applying CBT to a woman with depression

Joan's general practitioner referred her to the Community Mental Health Team. She had been complaining of ongoing and persistent depressive symptoms: low mood, tearfulness, poor appetite, poor sleep, and relationship difficulties with her husband. Joan thought her problems had arisen following the birth of her latest baby. She was not keen to use antidepressants and the GP requested the team assess Joan and if possible, offer appropriate treatment.

Community Mental Health Team assessment

A community psychiatric nurse and an occupational therapist from the Community Mental Health Team visited Joan (aged 29) at her home. The following is a summary of their assessment.

Presenting problem

At the assessment interview Joan described low mood, increased irritability, difficulty carrying out simple tasks, reduced libido, reduced memory, anhedonia (loss of pleasure), reduced concentration and reduced energy levels. She was very tearful when talking about her problems. She expressed some fleeting suicidal ideas but had no plans to act on them as she felt she was 'too much of a coward'. She denied that she wanted to harm herself. She also had somatic problems such as disturbed sleep; waking early in the morning without feeling refreshed. Her appetite was poor but she had not lost weight. In fact she had gained a little weight due to occasional binge eating. She felt that she was no longer in control of her life and had no time for herself with the pressures of full-time employment, children and housework. Her reluctance to take antidepressants was due to being unsure of the benefits.

History of presenting problem

Joan felt her problems started following the birth of her son Robert, her second child, a year ago. She felt that her mood was low and remembered feeling the same way after the birth of her daughter, Sarah, three years ago but she had not received help or treatment.

Past psychiatric history

Joan said she had never suffered from a mental health problem before but she had been aware of not feeling her usual self after the birth of her first child, Sarah.

Family history

Joan was aware that her maternal grandmother had been treated with ECT but was not sure why. Her grandfather suffered from senile dementia.

Background information

Joan was born in Newcastle. She was a middle child with an older sister and younger brother. The family moved around due to her father's job as an accountant. When Joan was two years old the family moved to Nigeria. Two years later, they returned to England and after a further four years they moved to Scotland where they had remained. She described herself as having been a shy child who tried to be liked by other children and was scared of criticism. She passed her exams at school and went to college where she graduated with a Diploma in Business Studies. She has been married for seven years. Her husband was a social worker and was described as being emotionally supportive. She worked full time as an administrator at a local health centre and had just returned to work following maternity leave but felt unable to cope and went on sick leave. Joan was ambitious and wanted to advance professionally but was frustrated that she did not have the higher business management qualification required to do so. She had a highly demanding workload with responsibility for operational management of the health centre and she regularly took work home. Due to some changes at work, there was a possibility that Joan could be redeployed or made redundant. The work performance of staff in the health centre was undergoing appraisal. Joan believed that her colleagues in the administrative team underperformed and she thought she was expected to do additional work to compensate for this.

Mental state

She appeared very low and was at times tearful but easily engaged in conversation. Her speech was fluent and articulate and she established good eye contact during the assessment interview.

Impression and action plan

The team's impression was of a 29-year-old woman with a diagnosis of depression who was willing to engage with services. A risk assessment was carried out and the team were confident that there was a low suicidal risk. The plan was to give advice and a course of antidepressant medication. In addition, it was recommended that Joan be taught problem-solving skills and receive cognitive–behavioural therapy.

Formal assessments

These were as follows:
- International Classification Disease (WHO 1992) – score F3: this indicated a mood (affective) disorder. (See Box 4.1.)

- Global Assessment of Function (Endicott et al 1976) – score 60, indicating moderate symptoms and generally functioning with some difficulty.
- Beck Depression Inventory (Beck & Steer 1987) – score 27, indicating a moderate level of depression.

Cognitive–behavioural therapy (CBT) sessions

First appointment

In the first CBT session, the therapist aimed to assess the relationship between thoughts, feelings, behaviours and physical symptoms and begin to formulate the case. Within this first appointment it was also important to establish a collaborative rapport that maximizes the patient's engagement in the process of therapy and introduce the CBT model.

When the therapist greeted Joan in the waiting area, she noticed that Joan was sitting on the edge of her seat, hunched forward, staring downwards and nervously winding her scarf around her hands. The therapist took Joan into her clinic room and explained what Joan could expect from the session. She asked Joan to describe her problems and concerns. She found Joan to be very negative about herself; she described herself as having 'always been shy' and lacking in confidence, particularly when getting to know people. She considered herself to be a 'terrible mother' and was concerned that her feelings for her husband had lessened. She also thought that her parents did not care about her. Joan told the therapist that she had decided to go off sick following an incident at home when she had lost her temper and had used excessive force while trying to bath her daughter who was being uncooperative. She was very distressed about her inability to control her daughter's behaviour and upset at her own aggressive behaviour.

Following Joan's description of her problems, the therapist described the CBT model and explained how it might be helpful to Joan. When 'socializing' Joan to the model it was important to use a recent situation when there had been a definite and marked change in Joan's feelings. This would help enable the therapist and Joan to identify the links between thoughts, feelings and behaviour. The following extract demonstrates how the therapist did this:

T: *I have told you a little about the theory behind cognitive–behavioural therapy and would like to help you understand how it relates to you and your situation. It would help both of us to look more closely at the situation you have just told me about that has distressed you. Would that be OK? [Joan nods in agreement.] It will give us both a clearer idea about the things that are going on that are making you feel so bad. So let's start by thinking about the situation you were in – you were bathing Sarah and she refused to get out of the bath – was it just you and Sarah that were there?*

J: *Yes – John was washing the dishes. Normally I like to do the children's baths. On that evening, I was tired and couldn't be bothered. Sarah had refused to have a bath at first. Then when she did eventually get in the bath, she was playing with her dolls and she didn't want to come out. It sounds awful but all I thought about was finishing the bath so that I could get her to bed and sit down in front of the telly and have a glass of wine.*

59

T. So what time was this – early evening – after teatime?

J. No, it was a bit later – we were late making dinner that evening – it was really past Sarah's bedtime.

T. OK. So you're bathing Sarah later than you should be and you are tired. How else did you feel?

J. Very low and irritated with Sarah.

T. I understand you felt low after a day at work, getting the tea ready and then putting Sarah to bed – it's a lot to fit in before you can sit down and rest. What went through your mind when you felt like this?

J. I thought, 'I wish Sarah would just get out of the bath when I ask her. She should be in bed by now. I am knackered. I want to sit down. This always happens to me. I can't get her to do as she's told and she is so cheeky. I don't like the way she is talking to me. If I was a good mother I could get her out of the bath'.

T. When you had these thoughts, how did you feel?

J. I started to get really angry with her.

T. So you had these negative thoughts and felt angry, what happened – did you do anything?

J. I stood up and got a towel and held it out to her for ages and kept saying 'Come on, out you get!' Then I just lifted her out, but really roughly. When I was drying her I really rubbed her too hard. I know I hurt her because she cried and then I felt like crying too. I just thought that I am a rotten mother. I can't do it.

T. I know this is really distressing for you, but this is actually a really good example that will show how CBT can help. Can I show you a sheet I have been filling in while you have been talking, it illustrates how all these things link together. [Joan is shown the 5 Areas Assessment – see Figure 4.1.]

T. When you have these negative thoughts about not being a good mother – how do you feel?

J. I feel very down. Low.

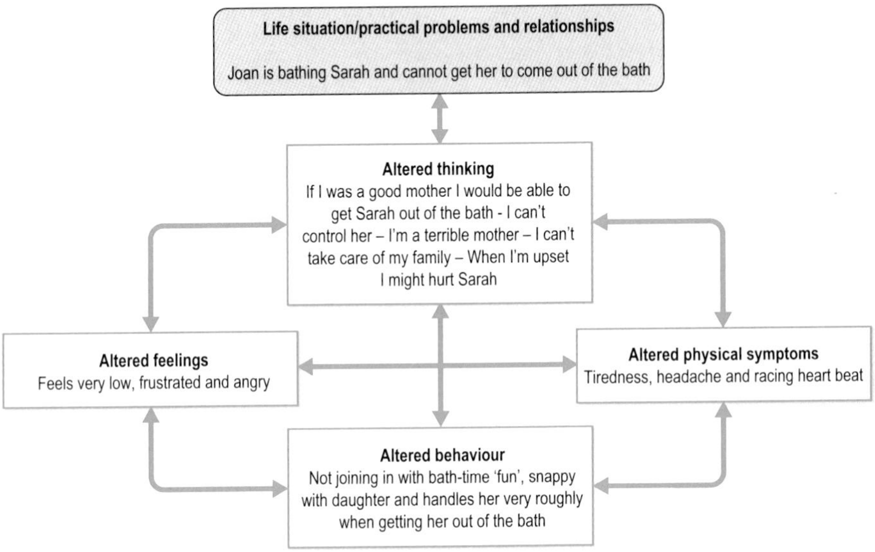

Life situation/practical problems and relationships

Joan is bathing Sarah and cannot get her to come out of the bath

Altered thinking

If I was a good mother I would be able to get Sarah out of the bath - I can't control her – I'm a terrible mother – I can't take care of my family – When I'm upset I might hurt Sarah

Altered feelings

Feels very low, frustrated and angry

Altered physical symptoms

Tiredness, headache and racing heart beat

Altered behaviour

Not joining in with bath-time 'fun', snappy with daughter and handles her very roughly when getting her out of the bath

Figure 4.1 ● Joan's initial five areas assessment.

T. Sometimes people when they are down are more likely to look at the negative side of things and be really hard on themselves. Do you tend to do that?

J. Yes. John says I'm like the person who always thinks that the bottle is half empty – not half full.

T. Looking at this, it seems that when you are tired, low and irritable, you tend to think very negatively about yourself. Is this true?

J. Yes but I have never really looked at things that way.

T. There also seems to be a link between your thoughts and feelings and what you do. It appears in the example you gave me that you are more likely to detach from Sarah and get irritable with her in these circumstances. You see how these things seem linked – your thoughts, feelings, behaviours?

J. I think so.

T. This way of looking at things helps in understanding why problems get us so down and it helps us decide what we are going to do about it. There is a link between how we feel, *think and act. We can look more closely at your thoughts and evaluate them as they may be affected by your mood rather than representing how things really are. It's how we judge or evaluate things that upset us, rather than how they are in themselves. Are they really true facts or is it how we interpret them? We can look at the things you are doing and think about different ways to deal with situations. We can do all this together and think about things that you can try out. I can tell you more about this in future sessions.*

This extract shows how the therapist asked questions that helped Joan identify her thoughts, feelings and actions. She summarized and repeated Joan's answers to confirm her understanding of what Joan had said. She empathized with Joan's feelings because it was important that Joan regarded the therapist as being non-judgemental. The therapist tried to normalize Joan's experience by letting her know that it is common for people with depression to have these thoughts and feelings. She also explained to Joan that there are interventions that would be helpful. The therapist's aim was for Joan to feel understood and to engender a sense of hopefulness and optimism that therapy might be helpful to her.

The therapist finished the session by explaining to Joan that she was expected to take work away from sessions and to try things out to see if they might be helpful. She gave Joan an 'Overcoming Depression' workbook (Williams 2001), which gave more information on the symptoms of depression, and asked her to fill in the first self-help exercise to increase her awareness of her thoughts, feelings, behaviours and physical symptoms.

By the end of the session the therapist has sufficient information to reach a tentative formulation of Joan's problems.

Initial formulation

A **critical early upbringing** and parental focus on achievement predisposed Joan to be vulnerable to depression. Joan's unhelpful thinking may have been **activated** when her performance at work was scrutinized and questioned, and redundancy considered. Joan **believed** that she would be exposed as a failure and this fear was applied to other major areas of her life, such as her role as a mother and relationship with her husband. For example, Joan had thought such as 'my boss thinks I am a failure', 'I am a rotten mother' and 'my husband does not care for me'. All her unhelpful thoughts are reinforced by the way she **processes information.** She has a negative thinking bias and tends to select certain negative aspects and uses this to interpret the whole situation. These thoughts link very powerfully to her **feeling** where she is low in mood and irritable. When she feels like this she can behave in unhelpful ways such as withdrawing from her daughter and focusing on unpleasant tasks. She avoids pleasure which increases how bad she feels. Joan had some **occupational dysfunction** due to her depression. **Her volition subsystem** is affected in that she has low levels of interest and a sense of personal causation; she feels out of control. Her **habituation subsystem** has become dominant with routines and habits being the main driver in her occupational behaviour. There is an obvious lack of pleasure in her life. Her **performance sub-system** is affected not through lack of skills but because she does not value her skills. Disturbance in each of these areas has led to conflict and a reduced ability to perform the **tasks** and **activities** that are required for her major occupational **life roles** as wife, mother and her work as an administrator.
(See Chapter 2 for further discussion around MOHO.)

Session 2

Although therapists may conceptualize a patient's problems within a specific model of therapy, the patient is unlikely to have knowledge about this model. The patient may therefore need some time to understand the model of therapy. It is important to keep 'socializing the patient to the model' whilst assessing the patient.

In the second session of therapy, the therapist asked Joan what she wanted to discuss that day and placed this on an agenda for that session. Using an agenda helps to keep the session focused on the main problems and issues that are relevant to the patient. Joan wanted to discuss the information booklet she had read. She said she had identified with the example of the woman with depression and was relieved to find that other people felt the same way. She had not appreciated how much depression had an impact on her life. She had completed the self-assessment and had also been thinking about her relationship with her husband. She thought that her husband might also be depressed as he had a lot of stress at work. She was concerned that they were 'unable to care for each other'.

The therapist noticed that Joan had developed a vicious circle of behaviour whereby she focused only on tasks that needed to be done and avoided pleasurable activities, including pleasure time with her children (see Figure 4.2). Joan did not appreciate that this may have contributed to maintaining her problems as she had beliefs that 'it's good to be active and get things done' and had very little insight into how having little pleasure had affected her. The therapist added this to her formulation.

The therapist shared a brief version of her formulation.

T: You have had some very strong early messages in your upbringing that have made you very sensitive to people assessing and judging your performance. It sounds like the situation you are facing at work is very stressful and has brought about changes in the way you feel, think and the things that you do. These changes are caught up in a vicious circle that keeps all your symptoms going. It is very common for people with depression to start thinking in a particular way. It's as if you have on a pair of dark glasses and can only see the negative side of things. Thoughts like 'I am a rotten mother' make you feel

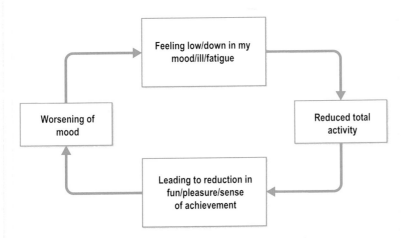

Figure 4.2 ● Joan's vicious circle of behaviour.

*very depressed and this can then result in you focusing on the housework and
withdrawing from Sarah. Roles that you have been comfortable with and enjoyed (for
example being a mother and wife) in the past are now a source of great stress. You are
focusing on the things you feel you have to do and have very little in your day that can
give you pleasure. Let's start with trying to change that.*

The therapist decided to take a behavioural approach, encouraging Joan to fill in
a typical day/weekly activity schedule and experiment with whether she was happier
when she was active, experiencing pleasure and achieving things.

Sessions 3–5: Increasing pleasurable activities

Each of the following sessions began by reviewing an activity schedule (see Box 4.2) or
a task that Joan had agreed to complete. This helped the therapist and Joan identify
past pleasurable and valued activities. Before the children were born, Joan had been
active, and had enjoyed cycling and swimming with friends. They both noted that Joan

---

Box 4.2

Joan's example of a typical day

Sometimes when people become unwell they lose structure to their day and this can
lead to losing touch with friends and not looking after yourself. In order to try and
change this we would like you to describe a typical day in your life.

Day and date	Activity (include everything you do)	Pleasure 0 = No pleasure 10 = maximum pleasure	How much of a sense of achievement did it make you feel
6–7 AM	In bed difficult to get up	0	0
7–8 AM	Get up and start getting Robert & Sarah ready for school and nursery	4	4
8–9 AM	Give kids their breakfast and take Robert to school then Sarah to nursery	4	4
9–10 AM	Go home and tidy up breakfast	3	3
10–11 AM	Have coffee alone	5	4
11–12 PM	Do some laundry	3	3
12–1 PM	"		

Time	Activity		
1–2 PM	"		
2–3 PM	Collect Sarah from nursery	4	3
3–4 PM	Collect Robert from school	4	3
4–5 PM	Homework with the kids	3	6
5–6 PM	Prepare family meal	3	3
6–7 PM	John home from work, he has had a bad day. Give family their dinner.	3	3
7–8 PM	Daughter refuses to finish dinner. Bathing daughter and getting her ready for bed	3	2
8–9 PM	Bedtime story	3	2
9–10 PM	Watch television with John and drinking with husband	6	3
10–11 PM	"		
11–12 PM	"		
12–1 PM	Go to bed	4	2

Scale:

0	5	10
No pleasure/ achievement	**Feel OK**	**Maximum pleasure/ achievement**

Review the day you have described and think about the answers to the following questions.

Do you think you make good use of your time? How much time is spent on pleasurable activities? Do you get a strong sense of achievement from the things you do? What do other people think about the way you spend your time?

Considering these answers – is there anything you would like to do differently? Write it in the box:

> My day is full of drudgery and tasks. I have no fun. I would like to do more with my friends

Sometimes when people become unwell they lose interest in things they used to enjoy or it is difficult to get going and do things. Having things that you enjoy in you life makes it easier to keep active. Do you have things that you enjoy doing?

What do you do?	Why do you like it?	How often do you do it?
Seeing friends	Good chat	Can't remember the
Cycling	Keeps me fit	last time
Doing things with the family when they behave	Fun	Never

Are there things that you used to be interested in but have stopped doing?

If so – list them	Why are you not doing them now?
Cycling and swimming Going visiting friends Going out clubbing Going out with husband to pictures or for a meal	Too much effort I feel let down by them Can't arrange babysitters "

Some people have things they think they are good at, what are you good at?

I was quite sporty at school

What sort of things are you not so good at?

I don't like being the centre of attention

Sometimes people feel uncomfortable when changes are made to their day. If changes are made to your routine how do you react?

There is rarely a change but sometimes the kids get sick at school – I just have to deal with it

Sometimes people feel they do not have control of their lives. Other people may be taking charge or you may find it difficult to make decisions. Do you feel in control of your life?

No ✓   Yes ☐

Give examples:

I can't do anything like I used to – I used to be very organized now just lose time

Physical problems can affect daily activities, for example lack of energy or lack of muscle strength. Are there any physical problems that affect your daily activities?

No ✓   Yes ☐

rated achievement lower as the day went by, and any activities that might had given her a sense of achievement earlier in the day were given progressively lower ratings. This change in the value assigned to her rating of activity possibly indicated a negative thinking bias. They agreed that there was an overall lack of pleasure in Joan's life that had become overly task-orientated with childcare. There was little time for herself in the day and clearly there was a need to reintroduce more pleasurable activities. Several patterns were observed such as Joan becoming stressed getting the children ready and out of the home in the morning. This appeared to start with Joan having difficulty getting up from bed. She lay in bed until the last minute then she would try to 'rush the children'. It was decided to reintroduce activities, broken down into step-by-step action plans. For example, Joan was to try to re-establish cycling with friends at quiet times and build up to using off-road cycling tracks. The work that Joan agreed to carry out between sessions would put these plans into action.

By the end of Session 3 the therapist and Joan were able to set some initial goals for therapy:
- Increase awareness of the thoughts Joan has about Sarah and the impact they have on her depression.
- Increase the pleasurable activities in Joan's life.

Sessions 6–7: Increasing awareness of negative thoughts

The therapist used dysfunctional thought records (Greenberger & Padesky 1995) to focus on increasing Joan's awareness of the impact of her negative thoughts. The most effective way to do this was to look at a specific time when Joan felt particularly low. This resulted in both her children and her husband John being regular topics for discussion in sessions (see example in Table 4.1).

Table 4.1 • Joan's negative automatic thoughts

1. Situation	2. Moods	3. Automatic thoughts (images)
At home with Sarah and she asks if she can have a friend over to visit	Feel really down Panicky and irritable 90%	I can't cope with having her friend over The kids never do what I say I'm a terrible mother They will make a terrible mess in the house No-one will help me to clear it up

Joan was encouraged to look at specific situations and identify her thoughts, feelings, physical symptoms, and behaviour. She was asked to rate her emotions as a percentage (feeling low 90%) and look for negative automatic thoughts (NATs).

Together, they identified that Joan was thinking in unhelpful ways that either lowered her mood or made her feel anxious – she tended to focus on the negative in a situation, would mind-read what other people thought of her, would make catastrophic predictions about how her children would 'turn out' and would ruminate on personal standards she had set such as 'I'll need to do the washing/ironing/clean the curtains'. Looking at the impact of these thoughts identified that she had begun to 'withdraw into herself' and that this was also unhelpful.

Joan frequently had a 'fantasy' image of herself being on her own sitting in a favourite holiday spot with no children and no husband placing demands on her. This reminded her of a time before she was married when she and her then boyfriend had temporarily split up – it had annoyed her husband that it took Joan two months to identify she wanted to be with him. The therapist was able to link this fantasy with Joan feeling vulnerable in her relationship with her husband.

Session 8: Review of main goals of therapy

This session focused on reviewing Joan's remaining goals in therapy. The therapist shared the formulation she had developed. Joan became very tearful but agreed with it. She identified her remaining goals as:

- Improving her relationship with John
- Exploring a return to work

They agreed these were long-term goals for therapy and split them into medium- and short-term goals. Having had success in getting pleasurable activities back into Joan's life, both agreed to begin working on the unhelpful thinking patterns that had contributed to maintaining her problems (see Table 4.2).

Sessions 9–12: Challenging negative thoughts

Joan began to challenge some of the negative thoughts that contributed to her low mood (see Table 4.3). Joan identified the most powerful negative thought and tried to evaluate the evidence for and against this thought. It was difficult to identify evidence against the thought and both the therapist and Joan agreed a good way to do this was to think 'what would my friends say to me if they heard me say this?' Joan could see that there was another way of looking at her negative thoughts and came up with a more balanced conclusion. However, she did not always believe strongly in her new balanced conclusions. Nonetheless, she noticed that evaluating her thoughts, or looking at them in a different way, did make a difference to the way she felt.

Through using dysfunctional thought records Joan became increasingly aware of underlying themes in the content of her automatic thoughts. She became more aware of the impact of her childhood experiences with her parents on how she judged herself.

Table 4.2 ● Joan's remaining goals

Goal	Short term	Medium term
Improve relationship with husband	Plan regular time together with husband apart from children Plan each day to talk it over with each other	Notice impact of thinking on behaviour, feelings and physical symptoms Use model to recognize husband's stresses Explore images re alternatives to marriage
Return to work	Identify rights re return to work following sick leave absence Arrange to meet with boss Establish routine at home to enable return Examine financial requirements Discuss with husband impact of not returning to work full-time on lifestyle	Meet up with staff/colleagues and confront reasons for absence Negotiate more reasonable working arrangements – part-time

Table 4.3 ● Joan challenging negative automatic thoughts

4. Evidence that supports the negative automatic thought	5. Evidence that does not support the negative automatic thought	6. Alternative/ balanced thoughts	7. Rate moods now
I can never get Sarah to do what she is told	*I love Sarah and want her to be happy*	*Feeling low makes it difficult to face the demands*	50%
She is much cheekier when her friends are over	*I want her to have positive memories*	*Sarah makes but I am a good*	
I don't have the energy to tidy up the terrible mess	*My friends say the same thing about*	*mother and spending time*	
I lose my temper and shout at her	*their children*	*with her can be*	
It would be awful if I was upset when a friend visits	*Sarah is excited and happy when her*	*fun*	
I am too rough with Sarah	*friends visit because they don't visit often*	*40%*	
	I am making very negative predictions about how the visit would go		

She was able to identify that being brought up by parents who focused on achievement and success contributed to her setting high standards for herself. Her parents had spent little time with their children and had a tended to be judgemental of the children's behaviour. Joan, earlier in therapy, had identified a vicious circle where she focused on tasks that needed to be done, and avoided pleasurable activities for herself or quality time with her children and husband. She had started to re-evaluate her belief that 'it's good to be active and get things done', and appreciated that this belief may contribute to some of her problems. Joan noticed that believing thoughts such as 'I am a terrible mother' prevented her from letting her daughter Sarah have positive experiences with her. The lack of a close positive relationship with her mother may have been related to Sarah's disruptive behaviour.

Joan continued to use dysfunctional thought records to help her prepare for returning to work. She was aware of unhelpful thoughts related to work (see Table 4.4). There were two themes that predominated:

- Joan disliked being the focus of attention and was highly sensitive to the scrutiny of others. She paid particular attention to her colleagues' and boss's opinions of her and she actively sought out reassurance and feedback on her performance.
- Joan was often unable to assert herself at work and socially. She did not stand up for herself and avoided confrontation.

She also had behavioural patterns that were probably unhelpful to her ability to get on with others and contributed to her feeling stressed at work. She isolated herself

Table 4.4 ● Joan gathering and challenging negative automatic thoughts

1. Situation	2. Moods	3. Automatic thoughts (images)	4. Evidence that supports the negative automatic thought	5. Evidence that does not support the negative automatic thought	6. Alternative/ balanced thoughts	7. Rate moods now
Feeling undervalued at work and thinking of a conversation with my boss when I made a mistake with the words I used	Feel really anxious, panicky and depressed Angry with colleagues 90%	Oh no, I've made a mistake He'll think I am an idiot who can't speak properly My boss doesn't let me take charge of complex jobs If I were good at my job I would not make mistakes I keep remembering a situation when I made a costly mistake with some items ordered for the surgery I don't want to make a mistake again	I mix my words up a lot I always make mistakes I made an expensive mistake in the past My boss doesn't believe my explanation He thinks I can't do the job I feel like a wee girl in the headmaster's room getting a row I don't like being in a situation when I am not in control of my feelings His opinion matters to me Everybody is dominant over me	I don't always make mistakes Some of my work is commended My workload is higher than everyone else I don't know what my boss is thinking unless I ask him It's not the same situation as when I was at school My feelings are powerful but I can control them.	I am making too much of a simple mistake – a slip of speech does not mean I am bad at my job 55%	40%

from others at work, asked for more work, worked over coffee breaks and after hours, and was fastidious in her attention to detail.

Alternative conclusions to her unhelpful thoughts were obtained through looking at the evidence for and against her thoughts. Beliefs and assumptions such as 'If I were good at my job I would not make mistakes' are replaced with 'I am making too much of a simple mistake'.

Session 13: Final session

The final session focused on reviewing Joan's progress in therapy to help her to identify what had been helpful or unhelpful, and what 'new life rules' she could develop to help her maintain her progress. Joan could appreciate the value of keeping a record of her achievements, and having a review day when she stopped and took stock of all the things she has done that were acceptable to her or had given her pleasure. The therapist and Joan reviewed all the lessons learned from earlier sessions. Joan had brought to the session a list of life rules and jointly they had compiled 'new life rules'.

Joan's new life rules

- I know I tend to see the negative in everything – it would be helpful to challenge this with my thought records and positive event log.
- To be a good mother I also need to make time to enjoy myself.
- It is good to be active and get things done but not to the exclusion of pleasurable time for myself.
- I do not need to seek other people's opinions of my work. I can make an appraisal of my own work.

Occupational therapists and physiotherapists will recognize similarities between the approaches that they feel very comfortable with. For example:

- Working collaboratively with patients
- Breaking down activities and taking step-by-step approaches to overcome problems and behaviours
- Examining and understanding the impact that values and core beliefs have in maintaining problems.

However, there are characteristics of CBT that can increase the effectiveness of the occupational therapist and physiotherapist. Therapists work with a diverse range of skills and interventions, and value their flexibility and ability to be creative problem solvers. However, there is a danger that they can sometimes lose focus in sessions and drift from the original aims they have identified. This can have value to the individual but can also result in the therapist taking a longer period of time to achieve their goals. In addition to this they need to reflect on whether they are adequately sharing their problem-solving skills with patients or are creating dependence when patients are unable to creatively solve their problems themselves. CBT is an approach that is very structured and places an emphasis on 'guided discovery' and teaching people a structure and the skills that will help them work with their own problems.

Perhaps the greatest enhancement that CBT can make to the role of the occupational therapist or physiotherapist is in working with cognitions. Joan's case clearly illustrates the way in which her negative thoughts and core beliefs were preventing her from moving on and giving herself permission to 'take more time for herself'. The way in which a person thinks about themselves and their situation affects everything they do. When cognitions and thoughts are not tackled there is a danger that therapists are only scratching the surface of a problem and sometimes reinforcing the negative views people have about themselves.

CBT enables occupational therapists or physiotherapists to work with their core skills in a focused, structured approach that teaches people problem solving, step-by-step behavioural interventions, increased awareness of their cognitions and challenging the impact that they have on their lives.

 ## Key Messages

- Depression is common.
- Cognitive–behavioural therapy for depression has an extensive evidence base.
- Cognitive–behavioural therapy for depression can reduce relapse rates.
- Cognitive–behavioural therapy is a structured time-limited psychosocial therapy.

References

Akiskal H S 1986 A developmental perspective on recurrent mood disorders: a review of studies in man. Psychopharmacology Bulletin 22(3):579–586

American Psychiatric Association 1994 Diagnostic and statistical manual of mental disorders, 4th edn. Washington, DC

Beck A T, Steer R A 1987 Manual for Beck Depression Inventory. Psychological Corporation, San Antonio

Beck A T, Rush A J, Shaw B F et al 1979 Cognitive therapy of depression: a treatment manual. Guilford Press, New York

Blackburn I M, Moore R G 1997 Controlled acute and follow-up of cognitive therapy and pharmacotherapy in out-patients with recurrent depression. British Journal of Psychiatry 171: 328–334

Blackburn I M, Eunson K M, Bishop S 1986 A two year naturalistic follow-up of depressed patients treated with cognitive therapy, pharmacotherapy, and a combination of both. Journal of Affective Disorders 10:67–75

Blacker C V R, Clare A W 1987 Depressive disorder in primary care. British Journal of Psychiatry 150:737–751

Burt V K, Stein K 2002 Epidemiology of depression throughout the female life cycle. Journal of Clinical Psychiatry 63(suppl 7):9–15

Crisp A H 2000 Changing minds: every family in the land. An update on the College's campaign. Psychiatric Bulletin of the Royal College of Psychiatry 24:267–268

Davidson K M, Connery H 2003 A Scottish survey of attitudes to depression in older and younger adults. Journal of Mental Health 12:505–512

Elkin I, Shea M T, Watkins, J T et al 1989 National Institute of Mental Health treatment of depression collaborative research program: general effectiveness of treatments. Archives of General Psychiatry 46:971–982

Elkin I, Gibbons R D, Shea M T et al 1995 Initial severity and differential treatment outcome in the National Institute of Mental Health treatment of depression collaborative research program. Journal of Consulting and Clinical Psychology 63:841–847

Endicott J, Spitzer R L, Fleiss J L et al 1976 The global assessment scale: a procedure for measuring overall severity of psychiatric disturbance. Archives of General Psychiatry 33(6):766–771

Evans M D, Hollon S D, DeRubeis R J et al 1992 Differential relapse following cognitive therapy and pharmacotherapy for depression. Archives of General Psychiatry 49:802–808

Feldman E, Mayou R, Hawton K et al 1987 Psychiatric disorder in medical inpatients. Quarterly Journal of Medicine 63:405–412

Giles D E, Jarrett R B, Biggs M M et al 1989 Clinical predictors of recurrence in depression. American Journal of Psychiatry 146(6):764–767

Greenberger D, Padesky C A 1995 Mind over mood: change how you feel by changing the way you think. Guilford Press, New York

Hollon S D, DeRubeis, R J, Evans M D et al 1992 Cognitive therapy and pharmacotherapy for depression: singly and in combination. Archives of General Psychiatry 49:774–781

Keller M B, Klerman G L, Lavori P W et al 1984 Long-term outcome of episodes of major depression: clinical and public health significance. Journal of the American Medical Association 252:788–792

Klein D F, Ross D C 1993 Reanalysis of the National Institute of Mental Health treatment of depression collaborative research program general effectiveness report. Neuropsychopharmacology 8:241–251

Kupfer D J 1991 Long-term treatment of depression. Journal of Clinical Psychiatry 52(suppl 5):28–34

Jacobson N S, Hollon S D 1996 Cognitive-behaviour therapy versus pharmacotherapy: now that the jury's returned its verdict, it's time to present the rest of the evidence. Journal of Consulting and Clinical Psychology 64:74–80

McLean P D, Hakstian A R 1979 Clinical depression: comparative efficacy of out-patient treatments. Journal of Consulting and Clinical Psychology 47:818–836

Murray C J, Lopez A D 1996 The global burden of disease: a comprehensive assessment of mortality and disability from diseases, injuries and risk factors in 1990 and projected to 2020. Harvard University Press, Cambridge, MA

Paykel E S, Hart D, Priest R G, 1998 Changes in public attitudes to depression during the defeat depression campaign. British Journal of Psychiatry 173:519–522

Posternak M A, Miller I 2001 Untreated short-term course of major depression: a metaanalysis of outcomes from studies using wait-list control groups. Journal of Affective Disorders 66(2–3):139–146

Priest R G, Vize A R, Roberts A et al 1996 Lay people's attitudes to treatment of depression: results of opinion poll for defeat depression campaign just before its launch. British Medical Journal 313:858–859

Rush A J, Beck A T, Kovacs M et al 1977 Comparative efficacy of cognitive therapy versus pharmacotherapy in out-patient depression. Cognitive Therapy and Research 1:17–37

Scott, A I, Freeman C P 1992 Edinburgh primary care depression study: treatment outcome, patient satisfaction, and cost after 16 weeks. British Medical Journal 304:883–887

Scott J, Palmer S, Paykel E et al 2003 Use of cognitive therapy for relapse prevention in chronic depression: cost effectiveness study. British Journal of Psychiatry 182:221–227

Shea M T, Elkin I, Imber S D et al 1992 Course of depressive symptoms over follow-up. Findings from the National Institute of Mental Health Treatment of depression collaborative research program. Archives of General Psychiatry 49:782–787

Solomon D A, Keller M B, Leon A C et al 2000 Multiple recurrences of major depressive disorder. American Journal of Psychiatry 157:229–233

Williams C 2001 Overcoming depression – a five areas approach, rev. edn. Arnold, London

WHO 1992 The ICD-199210 classification of mental and behavioural disorders: clinical descriptions and diagnostic guidelines. World Health Organization, Geneva

Cognitive–behavioural therapy for anxiety

George E Ralston

5

Introduction

Anxiety, fear, stress and worry are concepts everyone can relate to. We have all experienced these emotions at various points in our lives. In fact, anxiety is the only psychological problem that all of us can directly relate to through personal experience. Of course, not all our experiences are at problematic or diagnosable levels. However, we have all had anxiety as a consequence of a job interview, a trip to the dentist, a first date or some other everyday life experience. Anxiety, then, is a normal and common emotional response to stress or perceived threat.

However, this 'normal and common' response is now recognized as a major challenge in many ways. For example, it is estimated that approximately 20 billion euros per year are lost to job-related anxiety or stress. Stress is now the biggest cause of absenteeism, exceeding the previous most common problem presentation of 'chronic pain'.

There is a qualitative difference between the common levels of anxiety (which are often a reaction to environmental factors) and clinically recognized anxiety disorders, where the anxiety is experienced at greater intensity and has increased duration. It may be magnified or ameliorated by places, situations and individuals. Unlike everyday presentations of anxiety such conditions are very often significantly debilitating and may be chronic and longstanding.

Types of anxiety

DSM IV-TR identifies a number of anxiety disorders (American Psychiatric Association 1994). These are:

- *Specific phobia* (formally known as simple phobia). Here the main theme is significant and persistent anxiety in relation to a specific object or situation. Subtypes are: animal type (e.g. spiders), natural environment type (e.g. storms), blood injection-injury type, situational type (e.g. tunnels, lifts) and other type (e.g. choking or vomiting). Contact with or experience of the phobic object or situation ('stimuli') will lead to an immediate anxiety reaction. Further, the person recognizes that the fear is greater than it should be. They will subsequently avoid situations likely to lead to exposure to the feared stimuli and this is likely to have an adverse impact on their quality of life.

- *Social phobia* (also known as social anxiety). The main features here are a fear of one or more social situations where the individual worries that they will act in a way that is judged negatively by those around them. As with specific phobia, exposure to the social situations will almost inevitably lead to an anxiety response. The fear is recognized as excessive for the social situation and in turn is avoided if possible. As with all the anxiety conditions the person's quality of life is subsequently impaired.

- *Generalized anxiety disorder (GAD).* Here the sufferer will have significant worry and anxiety on most days and the worries will cover a range of events or activities. The GAD sufferer will find it impossible to control their worry and will experience a range of physical symptoms including muscle tension, sleep disruption and difficulties concentrating. These worries will also impair everyday functioning.

- *Panic disorder without agoraphobia.* Panic attacks involve an experience of fear which includes a range of symptoms including palpitations, sweating, trembling, chest pain, nausea and fear of losing control. The person with this condition will experience these symptoms on a recurrent basis; they will worry about having further attacks; they will be very concerned about the meaning of further attacks but they will not experience agoraphobia.

- *Panic disorder with agoraphobia.* In this condition the person experiences the above, but in addition suffers from agoraphobia. Here the sufferer will be fearful of being in places where they perceive they cannot easily escape. The person with agoraphobia typically worries about being in shops, queues, hairdressers, buses, trains and other enclosed places. As such they will avoid these situations.

- *Obsessive–compulsive disorder (OCD).* The central features here are repeated obsessions and/or compulsions. The obsessions are thoughts and images that the person experiences as intrusions in their everyday life. These cause significant levels of distress. These take many forms but the most common revolve around fears of contamination, doubts about actions or inactions, safety focus and/or sexual imagery. The associated compulsions occur as a way of reducing the anxiety created by the intrusive obsessions. Compulsions also take many forms. These include: repeated washing in relation to contamination fears; checking of electrical appliances in relation to fears of risk; and internal compulsions (alternative thoughts) to deal with negative imagery.

- *Post-traumatic stress disorder (PTSD).* Here the person has been exposed to an event which is beyond normal experience. This event is traumatic and leads to symptoms associated with re-experiencing the event by way of intrusive images, upsetting dreams, reliving the experience and distress when exposed to triggers associated in some way with the original traumatic experience. Coupled with these intrusive symptoms are avoidance phenomena. Here the person will avoid thoughts, feelings and conversations relating to the experience, they will avoid places associated with the event, they may be unable to remember certain elements of the experience, feel detached from others and find their emotional range is restricted. A final set of symptoms include heightened arousal which can lead to disturbed sleep, irritability, difficulty concentrating, hypervigilance and heightened startle response.

Prevalence

Research studies provide different prevalence figures for these disorders. Kessler et al (1994) in a US study suggests a lifetime prevalence for specific phobia of 11.3%. Wells et al (1989) found an estimate of 2.6% for social phobia. However, Sanderson et al (1990) has estimated that as many as 18% of those who request treatment in anxiety disorder clinics may have social phobia. In terms of GAD, the American Psychiatric Association suggests there is a lifetime prevalence rate of 5%. Data from Reich (1986) suggests the six-month prevalence for agoraphobia could be as high as 6% and for panic disorder 3%.

Obsessive–compulsive disorder estimates vary significantly, probably because there is a recognized under-reporting of this condition. Estimates vary from 1.5% by the Epidemiologic Catchment Area survey (ECA) and 3% by Oakley-Brown (1991). The ECA study suggests that only 34% of people with this condition report their symptoms to a health professional. Many studies have shown that the OCD sufferer will often go for years without disclosing this problem. Studies have found that half of those afflicted by OCD are female (Rasmussen & Tsuang 1986).

With PTSD, while general population estimates sit at around 1.3% (Davidson et al 1991), estimates relating to particular traumas can be significantly higher. Curran et al (1990) estimates that 50% of survivors of the Enniskillen bombing in Ireland had symptoms of PTSD; Kilpatrick et al (1987) found that 57% of women in a community sample who had been raped developed PTSD at some point in their life.

Comorbidity

Interestingly, anxiety disorders are often considered mild or moderate problems and this view then extends to a belief that they are easily treated. This is illustrated by organization of service provision, where services for 'severe and enduring' mental health problems often exclude people with anxiety. This population often receives help in the form of time-limited self-help or group treatments rather than individual assessment and therapy. In fact, anxiety disorders are often persistent, chronic and significantly disabling. This is partly explained by the fact that anxiety disorders often present with comorbid difficulties. The most frequently occurring comorbid problems are with co-occurring depression with estimates as high as 28% (Brown et al 2001), substance misuse with estimates in PTSD being as high as 50% (Kessler et al 1995) and personality disorder with Reich et al (1987) suggesting between 40–63% of people with agoraphobia have associated personality disorders.

The high levels of comorbidity create significant challenges both for service commissioners and for therapists. For the latter, a recognition of the complexity of anxiety as a presenting condition may enable the therapist to pay particular attention to assessment and formulation. Taking time to consider these, as opposed to jumping headlong into an intervention, may pay dividends in the long term for the client's therapy. The assessment and formulation will enable a tailored CBT intervention for the client and will maximize the possibility of a successful outcome. For commissioners the challenge is not to see anxiety as a unidimensional disorder which can be swiftly and briefly treated by a range of qualified professionals. It needs to be viewed as a disorder which presents in various forms of complexity and which therefore requires a service to have the ability to respond with appropriate flexibility and sensitivity to individual presentations.

Context

While the physiotherapist or occupational therapist working in mental health settings will quickly be able to identify these anxiety-related conditions and associated comorbid difficulties, those working in other settings may witness anxiety in different forms. A likely presentation is the patient who is recovering from a physical health problem but who is held back by anxieties over their condition or their future. For example the patient who has suffered a stroke may be worried that they will not be able to do many of the everyday tasks they managed before. They may be anxious about the possibility of future strokes. The patient with chronic pain may be worried about the impact their pain may have on leisure activities they enjoy or their employment. A patient recently diagnosed with multiple sclerosis may have anxieties following information they have read about possible future difficulties with incontinence or sexual dysfunction.

Physiotherapists and occupational therapists find themselves working in a variety of settings and so this chapter will consider general principles in the treatment of anxiety through cognitive–behavioural means as opposed to individual treatment approaches to different conditions. However, for those interested in different models of anxiety and different treatments for the range of anxiety conditions then the work of Wells (1997) and Clark (1986) is recommended.

Cognitive model of anxiety

There are a variety of models of anxiety disorders and a number of cognitive theories. This chapter largely draws on the work of Beck and his colleagues (1985). It is this work that has been most widely researched and now drives much of our thinking about anxiety. Within Beck's model he argues that anxiety is created and maintained by:

- An overestimation of danger
- An overestimation of its impact
- An underestimation of personal ability to cope
- An underestimation of rescue factors.

Certainly, if one listens to those experiencing anxiety one will hear them suggesting the inevitability of some disaster occurring; of the consequences of this being catastrophic; of them 'not being able to cope' and rarely expressing the notion that others can help if necessary. Consider the following illustrative examples with Beck's four factors in mind:

- A client who has had a myocardial infarction has thoughts which indicate that they expect a future heart attack to be inevitable, that they will definitely die as a consequence, that they cannot do anything to prevent this and that no one can be a help.
- A client with OCD believes that they will definitely be contaminated by touching door handles, that this will lead to a terrifying physical reaction, that they will not be able to cope with the anxiety they have as they approach the door, and that no one will be able to help them deal with their distress.
- A client with a phobia of lifts thinks that going in a lift will inevitably mean it will break down and they will be trapped. If this were to happen they believe that this will be a 'disaster', they do not think they will be able to cope with the experience and they fail to acknowledge how easily they will be helped.

Central to Beck's writings is his notion of different levels of cognition. At the surface level we have negative automatic thoughts (NATs). NATs occur in verbal or imaginal form and are strongly held at the time they occur. They are automatic and negatively appraise or interpret events. These NATs are often linked to particular behavioural and emotional responses. Most of us when NATs are described very quickly become aware of their daily presence in our minds. We also become aware of hearing the spoken NATs of our friends and family. We hear them say things like:

- 'I'll fail this exam.'
- 'This interview will be torture.'
- 'I bet they will mess me around.'

NATs are reflective of the second of Beck's 'levels of cognition' which are the underlying assumptions and, at a deeper level, our constructs or beliefs. Assumptions are conditional statements of the 'If . . . then' form. For example, a person may say '**If** I show fear **then** people will think I'm weak and inferior', or '**If** I have these physical symptoms **then** I must have a serious illness'. Beliefs, on the other hand, are usually expressed as unconditional, definitive statements such as 'I am . . .'. For example, 'I am a failure'; 'I am inferior to others'; 'I am stupid' and 'I am weak'.

In the last few years it has been hypothesized (Wells 1997) that the content of assumptions and beliefs differs dependent on the anxiety disorder. For example, with panic disorder assumptions and beliefs about symptoms and bodily events are paramount, whereas in GAD beliefs tend to revolve around a self-view perpetuating an inability to cope and beliefs about the nature of worry per se. However, while the content of the appraisals and schema may differ in some respects with each disorder there are some things common to all. There are positive feedback cycles between cognition, symptoms and behaviour; dysfunctional appraisals; cognitive biases; and avoidance and safety behaviours.

The biases in the way information is processed are referred to as 'thinking error patterns' or 'cognitive distortions'. These include the following:

- *Selective attention.* Here a person will 'attend' to one aspect of a situation while ignoring other, often more relevant, information. This is comparable to attending to the corner of a picture while ignoring the whole painting or listening to one line of a song while ignoring the other verses.

- *Overgeneralization.* Here a person arrives at a conclusion to a wide range of events based on a single or very few incidents. For example, they may conclude that they are woeful at maths by recalling a single failed exam, or they may conclude they are inferior to others because they took three attempts to pass their driving test.
- *Black-and-white thinking.* Here a person is unable to think in shades of grey. Things are either perfect or awful; they have done a great job or a pitiful one.
- *Ignoring the positive.* Here a person will focus on the negative elements of a situation and/or themselves while ignoring the positives. For example, they may think about the mistake they made, while ignoring the many occasions when they have done something well. They may remember vividly the criticism they received while failing to recall the compliments they have had.
- *Catastrophizing.* Here a person creates thoughts or images in their mind of disproportionately negative outcomes. They may think that they will lose their job following a critical comment from their boss.

To illustrate how cognitive biases can maintain belief in negative interpretations, consider the example of the client who is in cardiac rehabilitation with his physiotherapist. He is being encouraged to build up his exercise programme and while doing this becomes aware of his increasing heart rate. He suddenly begins to sweat more, to notice his breathing is quickening and believes that he may be in danger of experiencing another heart attack. As a consequence of this experience he fails to carry out his exercise regimen between his appointments and starts to become more sedentary. In this example, we see 'selective attention' and 'catastrophizing'. He has focused in on physical sensations and then misinterpreted normal bodily reactions to exercise in a catastrophic fashion. Not surprisingly the outcome is ever heightening physical symptoms of anxiety and consequent avoidance or the employment of safety behaviours.

Schema or beliefs have often had their seeds sown when a person was growing up, early childhood and adolescence being particularly relevant periods. The beliefs they have about themselves, others and the world will be influenced by their interpersonal and other life experiences and their underlying character (Young et al 2003). The beliefs a person who is anxious characteristically holds relate to notions that the world is a dangerous place, that harm is likely to come to them, that their fate (which they are helpless to alter) may be a seriously negative one and that they are on their own in dealing with events.

The levels of cognition are important when working with those with anxiety. Targeting them can not only aid the client in understanding why they feel the way they do, but also why others in similar situations may not respond in the same way and how to make changes at each level to maximize the potential for lasting change.

Assessment – engagement

The first step in cognitive therapy for anxiety is assessment. As with all therapies the relationship between therapist and client is key. In the context of assessment it is critical. Engagement with the anxious patient will determine whether the person is able to be clear about the nature of their condition. It will also determine whether or not they are able to return for therapy and most importantly whether they can undertake the necessary steps in order to benefit from therapy. This is especially pertinent since a key component of therapy will be an expectation that the patient will challenge their current avoidance pattern and, over time, expose themselves to the very situations that currently cause them so much distress. How able they are to do this will often be determined by their own motivation and commitment but also by the relationship they have with their therapist. They need to have sufficient confidence and trust in this person to tackle the various scenarios that will face them. Further, the collaborative nature of cognitive–behavioural therapy (CBT) means that therapy is most likely to succeed when the patient is an active participant in the process. Engagement can facilitate how able a patient feels in participating in the therapy process.

Within the clinical interview the therapist must ascertain whether CBT is likely to be an appropriate therapy for this particular patient at this particular time. The therapist is examining the following:

Presenting problem: physiological symptoms; cognitive symptoms; behaviours; emotions; duration of episode; intensity; avoidance phenomena

Aetiological factors: first episodes; possible influences; employment history; relationship history; psychiatric history; psychological history

Coping abilities: internal coping abilities; external coping abilities; hobbies/ interests; alcohol and drug history

Possible assumptions

ABC analysis: antecedents; appraisals and beliefs; consequences; maintaining factors; worseners/improvers

History: upbringing; education experience

Current circumstances: occupation; living situation

Possible schema

Assessment – measures

A second key element of assessment for CBT is the employment of a variety of assessment measures. The reason for including these is twofold: initially, as a way of gathering further information on the nature of an individual's difficulties; secondly, these assessments enable the therapist and patient to monitor progress during therapy and at the end and during follow-up sessions. There are a variety of measures employed but the main ones are:

- BAI (Beck Anxiety Inventory): a 21-item self-report questionnaire rating the severity of anxiety a client is experiencing (Beck 1990).
- BDI II (Beck Depression Inventory): a 21-item self-report questionnaire rating the severity of depression a client reports (Beck 1996).

These are termed global scales as they measure generally how anxious and depressed a person may feel. More specific questionnaires targeted at individual conditions will also be used in CBT. Examples of these are:

- CBOCI (Clark-Beck Obsessive Compulsive Inventory): a 25-item self-report form which has two subscales, one for obsessions and one for compulsions. A total score is also calculated (Clark & Beck 2002).
- Fear Questionnaire: a 15-item questionnaire which explores the 15 most common presenting phobias. There are three subscores for agoraphobia, blood injury phobia and social phobia (Marks & Mathews 1979).
- SPS (Social Phobia Scale): a commonly used self-report scale focusing on fear of being observed by others. It is often employed with its companion scale, the Social Interaction Scale, which assesses one's anxiety level while interacting with others (Mattick & Clarke 1998).
- IES (Impact of Events Scale): allows clients to report their experience of avoidance of reminders about the trauma and the extent to which thoughts about the event come into their daily lives (Horowitz et al 1979).

Other assessment measures include patient ratings of their emotions and diaries/records of situations where anxiety is experienced.

Behaviour tests

Behaviour tests are an excellent way for the therapist to get a more objective view of events and can also help assess the client's own ratings of emotions and cognition content in a live situation. Such tests may include taking the agoraphobia sufferer outside and exploring the impact using the basic CBT model of emotions, physical symptoms, cognitions and behaviours. Of course such behavioural experiments elicit anxiety and need to be managed very carefully. Failure to do so is likely to prejudice the relationship with the therapist and may lead to a client dropping out of therapy prematurely.

82

Contraindications for treatment of anxiety

Clients with medical conditions such as cardiac disease, emphysema, epilepsy or severe asthma may be discouraged from carrying out certain CBT procedures such as hyperventilation. Others with psychosis may require assistance initially to stabilize their well-being before embarking on CBT for co-occurring anxiety. Clients who are regularly intoxicated may be helped by treatment for their addiction before considering tackling their anxiety disorder. The clinician needs to be aware that not every presenting person is suitable at that time for CBT. They may benefit from such an intervention later on; however, it is important not to embark on any treatment if there are doubts about its appropriateness or efficacy as this may lead to clients who are unsuccessful attributing failure to themselves rather than to the mistiming of the intervention. They may also prematurely conclude that CBT is not effective for them rather than attributing the failure to current adverse conditions in their lives which may be the real blocks to success.

Treatment

Socialization

Initial stages of treatment (including assessment) provide opportunities to socialize clients to the CBT model (Wells 1997). This is often carried out in a staged form to facilitate comprehension and recall, since presenting a schema-based formulation may be inappropriate for some clients or overwhelming to others. Initially, the emphasis may be on sharing examples of the links between emotions, cognitions, physical symptoms and behaviour. General examples and ones pertinent to the client are both helpful. Further, clients often require help in understanding their role in therapy. Those new to psychological therapy may not be familiar with the notion that they have an active role to play, that the therapist is not the sole expert in the room, that the therapist alone does not have all the answers and, finally, that any change made will be through the actions of the client themselves. This can seem strange and inhibiting initially to some individuals and very liberating and energizing to others. At this time it is also essential that clients are educated as to the format of each session, including agenda setting, shared goal setting and home-based tasks. The process of socializing can often make or break therapy. Taking time during this stage will lead to engagement in therapy and enable the therapist and client to work most effectively, enhancing the probability of a successful outcome.

As part of the initial socialization phase the therapist will also introduce information about the CBT model for the client's anxiety problem. It is often helpful to provide the client with information on their condition. This helps them see the connection between fear, anxiety and worry. It also leads onto an understanding of the links between cognition, emotion, physiology and behaviour. There are a plethora of resources about anxiety in different formats. It is the therapist's responsibility to match their client with the best information. This involves some assessment of their education level, motivation, and also some exploration of how they best learn.

The socialization phase should also be guiding the client to recognize some optimism about the treatment they are starting. This is aided by the information discussed and given to them, by the model as outlined with their individual profile and by the positive approach and optimism of the therapist.

Challenges in engagement

Of course CBT, as with all therapies, does not suit everyone. Inhibiting factors include the client thinking that the rationale does not fit with their internal view of their problem. Or the client may believe strongly that their problem is physical in nature and cause. The client may have difficulty in identifying their thought processes and imagery. Other clients struggle with elements of the therapy including record keeping and home-based work. Overcoming such challenges requires all the therapist's expertise; with a few they may need to accept CBT is not right for this person at this time, and alternatives may need to be explored.

The elements of the model are separated below in order to highlight the different techniques. As a therapist's experience develops, and through good supervision, the different elements become seamlessly integrated.

Treating the cognitive element

The cognitive element refers to the thoughts, images, assumptions and beliefs an individual holds. There have been a number of different approaches to tackling their dysfunctional aspects. This chapter will focus on two main areas, namely 'cognitive restructuring' and the 'management of worry'.

Cognitive restructuring

In cognitive restructuring an individual is helped to recognize the way their thinking influences their emotions, their physiology and their behaviour. First they must be helped to recognize their negative cognitive content, then they can learn a variety of ways of challenging it. Doing this effectively will lead to improved outcomes across the other elements in the model.

The first step is recognition. The most common method of identifying negative thoughts is by use of clinical interview and accompanying this with the use of a diary. In the clinical interview the cognitive–behavioural therapist will be able to guide the individual in identifying common negative cognitions. Between sessions the individual is encouraged to keep a record of episodes of negative thought content. This usually takes the form of a diary which details the situation that occurred, a description of the emotion this elicited and some rating of its strength, and then a written narrative of what was going on for the person cognitively. This may take the form of a distressing image, or a series of negative thoughts about themselves, their situation or the future.

This initial stage can be difficult for individuals, especially the recognition and description of the actual thoughts that go on in their mind. Individuals often find it far easier to describe the situation and the emotion they experienced. They are less adept at rating the level of their emotion, the recognition of the negative thoughts and their belief rating in these. Considerable work within the session going over past and current experiences will aid this process. This is especially helpful if there is an emotional shift within the session. If this occurs it will usually be representative of some negative thought that has just occurred for the individual. By checking out 'What went through your mind just then?' the therapist will gain live information on the type of thoughts that the person has and a great opportunity of helping them experience the cognitive model 'in person' and in the here and now.

Once the thoughts, images have been identified the therapist and the individual can now begin the process of 'restructuring' the cognitive content. One commonly employed technique here is referred to as the 'court room' technique. In a court of law a proposition is made: 'Mr X is guilty of crime Y'. Then evidence is presented which supports this proposition, followed by evidence that challenges this proposition. The same approach is taken with negative thoughts. The individual thought, assumption or belief is detailed and then evidence for and against this is examined.

For example, a person who suffers from panic disorder may have the negative automatic thought that the chest pain they have just began to feel is evidence that they are about to have a heart attack. Their role here is to examine the evidence for and against this thought. Evidence for may include knowledge they have that people who have heart attacks experience chest pain, they feel light-headed and then become dizzy. Evidence against this thought may be that they have had the identical feelings in the past and never experienced a heart attack, there is no family history of heart condition, the pain is more likely to reflect that they have indigestion, and so on.

This technique is immensely helpful. Before they learn how to do this clients are likely to have solely focused on the negative thought. It will rarely have any evidential support and this technique encourages the exploration of alternative evidence of which there is often a good deal.

Another helpful technique for undermining negative automatic thoughts is 'identifying cognitive errors'. Here the individual is enabled to see that their thinking has developed distinctive patterns which are referred to as cognitive errors. With anxiety, these habitual forms of thinking involve overestimating danger and underestimating coping abilities. Common thinking errors are outlined earlier in this chapter. Increased awareness of the thinking errors they have developed helps the individual recognize that it is this style of thinking which is causing them so much distress, not actual events in their lives. Recognition of these thinking errors and their habitual nature will help the client reduce the impact of the negative thoughts. When they encounter what is usually (for them) an anxiety-provoking situation they will be able to identify their habitual thinking errors, immediately undermining the potential impact of that situation.

A further technique that many clients find helpful is to ask themselves 'How would someone else think about this?'. The client's overestimation of danger does not often generalize to what they believe a significant other person in their life may think. Clients are asked to imagine how their therapist, their partner, parent or friend might think about the situation. This technique is simple but powerful as it gives the client a much-needed alternative perspective to balance against their negative thoughts.

'What if?' is a popular technique. Clients often do not actually take their thoughts to a logical ending. As such they are left with the negative emotion and a ruminating thought. By going to 'What if?' the client examines what might happen if their worst thought came true. So the person who has a negative thought about their work performance, when taken to its conclusion may have a more powerful negative thought such as 'I will lose my job'. By doing this the client often discovers that the feared outcome is extremely unlikely or that the feared outcome is something they can develop an action plan to manage and so the anxiety is significantly reduced.

A final technique relates to the frequency with which clients with anxiety underestimate their own ability to cope. A review of past experiences similar to those they are in or about to enter will provide convincing evidence to them that they can cope. This is far more powerful than therapist persuasion. Their own experience will be the convincing data in this test. It may even be helpful for clients to maintain a positive diary record wherein they record past successes. By regularly reviewing this they will improve their self-efficacy and increase the probability of successfully negotiating situations in the future.

Management of worry

The management of worry involves the development of 'worry time', a technique to 'contain' worry developed by Borkovec et al (1983). An anxious individual will often spend inordinate amounts of time worrying about some impending situation which may or may not take place. This is not productive time that involves an analysis of possibilities and the development of an action or problem-solving plan. It is in effect time spent unintentionally magnifying and intensifying their anxiety. This extended worry also generalizes their anxiety by linking new stimuli which create new associations with anxiety beyond those from the original experience. Using the worry-time technique, clients are encouraged to schedule a time for worry and to keep any worry to this time frame. The client identifies specific anxieties from a diary they have kept. A time and location is then agreed with the therapist considering these worries. When worry occurs beyond this time the client is actively encouraged to simply accept its appearance and to outline when it will be considered. The client then focuses their attention on what they are doing currently. When the worry time comes around they use the time to bring out their anxieties. The client is also actively encouraged to tackle the worry at this time through the use of the cognitive restructuring techniques outlined above.

Treating the physiological element

There are a variety of physical changes associated with anxiety. The physiological systems involved include the nervous system, the cardiovascular and respiratory functions and the gastrointestinal process. Heightened arousal is a key characteristic of anxiety. For many years it has been acknowledged that it is possible with training to influence these physiological reactions. A variety of methods have been developed for this, two of which are outlined here.

Deep progressive muscular relaxation

This form of relaxation was originally used by Jacobson (1929) and was first modified by Wolpe (1958). It has been widely used in a range of studies (e.g. Ost & Breitholtz 2000). Here the therapist teaches the client how to relax all the major muscle groups in their body through tensing and relaxing each muscle set. The client is then encouraged to practice both within and between therapy sessions. Deep progressive muscular relaxation is a skill and as such requires effort and discipline to achieve mastery in it. The client is encouraged to practice twice daily initially and then on a continued but less frequent basis. Practice through the use of an audio recording of the relaxation instruction can be very helpful for individual clients. Once the client has mastered the progressive muscular relaxation they are encouraged to practice parts of it in everyday situations such as being on the bus, standing in a queue or sitting at their work station. By practising in a variety of places their level of physical tension overall is greatly reduced. Further, when they need to utilize relaxation for a situation that is anxiety provoking, they will be better able to bring this skill into action as they have practised it effectively. In one version of relaxation clients are encouraged to work on a cue-controlled approach as a final phase. This involves using the word 'relax' to create the state of relaxation. The focus here is on breathing and exhaling with the word 'relax' in their mind. Clients repeat this for several minutes. Over time many clients, using this method, can relax very swiftly over a period of 2–3 minutes.

Diaphragmatic breathing

This is another form of relaxation which helps clients to deal with unpleasant physiological consequences of anxiety. Once again the therapist emphasizes the importance of practice in mastering this skill. The client is given information on breathing. They then place one hand on their abdomen and one on their chest. As they breathe they observe which hand moves. The client is then encouraged to relax and watch the slowing down of the movement in their abdomen. Once again the introduction of the word 'relax' can help the client focus their mind on the physical response they are experiencing.

Treating the behavioural element

The central goal in the behavioural element is to assist the client to expose themselves to previously avoided situations. If done correctly their anxiety will be extinguished and a change in cognitive content will ensue as the client will experience for themselves the absence of a catastrophic outcome and a recognition of their ability to cope with challenging situations.

In vivo exposure

Initially the therapist and the client develop a hierarchy of situations currently viewed as problematic. These are ranked in order of difficulty. The number of situations is less relevant than the need to have small steps in difficulty between them. Once these are identified the therapist and the client agree to tackle the first step on the hierarchy. Planning on how to deal with this is essential. The therapist and patient speculate on any potential challenges. This can include examining the anticipatory period in particular and suggesting probable cognitions that may occur and how the client is going to challenge these. In-session practice of such challenges can be very effective. The therapist may also encourage the client to manage the physiological response through relaxation, especially in this anticipatory period. If a client finds a step is too challenging initially they and the therapist together will modify this goal and find an in-between step. Progressively over time the client notices a reduction in their anxiety levels when tackling each situation. The co-occurring change in cognitions may also begin to manifest itself. Through this exposure their cognitions will alter to ones where they expect to be able to manage anxiety, where they believe anxiety is not catastrophic and where they are growing in confidence about being able to manage challenging situations.

Pleasurable activities

The measurement and enhancement of pleasurable activities is commonly part of the intervention within CBT for depression. However, there are therapists who also recognize the benefit of using this with anxiety. The presentation of anxiety often includes excessive worry which in turn reduces the client's participation in recreational and occupational activities. Encouraging the identification and planning of pleasurable activities will provide respite from ineffectual worry, providing an alterative focus for the client's attention.

Problem solving

A final behavioural approach is problem solving (Meichenbaum & Jaremko 1983). Clients are helped to see that they often encounter two difficulties when problem solving. That is they (a) view the problem in vague, general ways and (b) do not consider solutions that may help. Clients are encouraged to break problems down into discrete behavioural components. Thought sharing their way to solutions is the next stage. This stage involves client and therapist generating as many solutions as possible *without* examining their merits. Once a full list is generated, each solution is considered from a strengths and weaknesses position. An option is then selected, implemented and then reviewed. As well as helping the client create solutions this approach will also help build their expertise in thinking differently about problems in their life and to address realistic as opposed to catastrophic possibilities. In essence this approach can work in the same way as exposure, enabling clients to see for themselves that the predicted catastrophe will not occur and that they are able to cope with the challenges they face.

Dealing with relapse

As indicated earlier, treating anxiety problems can be a challenging and complex process. Many sufferers have long-standing and complex presentations. There are those who have been through therapy many times or who have tried different forms of help with mixed results. Relapse therefore is clearly an issue which needs to be considered.

The best time to begin considering relapse is before the end of the client–therapist sessions. Work conducted on relapse can prevent or forestall it. The therapist talks to the client about the possibility of relapse. This is framed in terms of slips, setbacks or minor recurrence of past symptoms. The client is encouraged to see this as a slip and not as a return to pre-existing levels of difficulty. The 'snakes and ladders' metaphor can be helpful here. The child's game illustrates for the client that they can slip as one does on a snake in this game but one does not go back to square one. The introduction of the possibility of relapse by the therapist, furthermore, gives permission for concerns about future 'slips' to be aired by the client, allowing the therapist to reinforce normalizing messages about a less than perfect future state, in which anxiety, sometimes quite intense, might recur. Indeed, even if the client slips down the longest snake, there is an assumption that they can work their way back up through the 'game' of anxiety management.

Clients are helped to understand that as they progress they will be less inclined to practice their new found skills. As such they become 'rusty' and less available when necessary. It can be this that leads to setbacks. They are therefore encouraged to plan 'reflection time'. This is a formal time set aside where they monitor their progress over that past week/month, using a series of self-addressed questions. How was my anxiety? What situations trigger anxious symptoms? What were my NATs? What techniques did I use? What others would have worked in this situation? Reflection time is clearly very beneficial. The client maintains their progress with such a focus, not expecting it to continue without ongoing effort. They also begin to see what techniques work, and further, it might encourage them to expand their repertoire.

Booster sessions are also very helpful in preventing relapse. Here sessions are planned with increasingly spaced time intervals. Between these sessions clients are expected to continue with their work and to be able to come to the booster session with a good description of what has gone well and why, as well as a review of less successful experiences, what the contributory factors were and on reflection what they might have done differently.

A final effective way of preventing relapse is enlisting the help of a family member who can act as a co-therapist. They are knowledgeable about their relative and the elements of their anxiety. The family member needs to be helped to gain a basic understanding of the interventions employed and a recognition of their role as 'coach', someone who encourages their relative to continue to use their new-found skills. The coaching role will benefit clients considerably.

Conclusion

Anxiety is a common emotional response which we can all relate to. A cognitive–behavioural model highlights the importance of the cognitive content of anxiety responses. Over recent years theorists have began to explore different models of anxiety and different interventions for anxiety disorders (Wells 1997, Clark 1986). This chapter has focused on the key elements of a cognitive approach to managing anxiety. The techniques outlined are by no means exhaustive but are intended to illustrate the particular elements and different approaches. A cognitive–behavioural therapist needs to be skilled and experienced at selecting the approach and integrating the techniques which will differ for different client presentations.

 ## Key Messages

- Anxiety is a well-recognized emotion.
- Anxiety disorders are costly to society in lost days at work and treatment costs.
- Anxiety manifests itself in a number of different types of disorders each with their own symptomology.
- There is a body of evidence for using CBT in the treatment of anxiety disorders.
- The different approaches in treating the cognitive, behavioural and physiological elements should be combined to provide an integrated treatment approach.

89

American Psychiatric Association 1994 Diagnostic and statistical manual of mental disorders, 4th edn. Washington, DC, Author

Beck A T 1990 Beck Anxiety Inventory. Psychological Corporation, San Antonio

Beck A T 1996 Beck Depression Inventory, 2nd edn. Psychological Corporation, San Antonio

Beck A T, Emery G, Greenberg R L 1985 Anxiety disorders and phobias: a cognitive perspective. Basic Books, New York

Borkovec T D, Wilkinson L, Folensbee R et al 1983 Stimulus control applications to the treatment of worry. Behaviour Research and Therapy 21:247–251

Brown T A, Campbell L A, Lehman C L et al 2001 Current and lifetime comorbidity of the DSM-IV anxiety and mood disorders in a large clinical sample. Journal of Abnormal Psychology 110:585–599

Clark D M 1986 A cognitive model of panic. Behavioural Research and Therapy 24:461–470

Clark D, Beck A T 2002 Clark-Beck Obsessive Compulsive Inventory. Manual, Psychological Corporation, San Antonio

Curran P S, Bell P, Murray G et al 1990 Psychological consequences of the Enniskillen bombing. British Journal of Psychiatry 156:478–482

Davidson J R, Hughes D, Blazer D G et al 1991 Post-traumatic stress disorder in the community: an epidemiological study. Psychological Medicine 21:713–721

Horowitz M, Wilner N, Alvarez W 1979 Impact of Event Scale: a measure of subjective stress. Psychosomatic medicine 40:209–218

Jacobson E 1929 Progressive relaxation. University of Chicago Press, Chicago

Kessler R C, McGonagle K A, Zhao S et al 1994 Lifetime and 12 month prevalence of DSM-III-R psychiatric disorders in the United States. Archives of General Psychiatry 51:8–19

Kessler R C, Sonnega A, Bromet E et al 1995 Post-traumatic stress disorder in the National Comorbidity Survey. Archives of General Psychiatry 52:1048–1060

Kilpatrick D G, Veronen L J, Saunders B E et al 1987 The psychological impact of crime: a study of randomly surveyed crime victims, Final report, Grant Number 84-IF-CX-0039. National Institute of Justice, Washington, DC

Marks I M, Mathews A M 1979 Brief standard self-rating for phobic patients. Behaviour Research and Therapy 1:263–267

Mattick R P, Clarke J C 1998 Development and validation of measures of social phobia scrutiny fear and social interaction anxiety. Behaviour Research and Therapy 36:455–470

Meichenbaum D S, Jaremko M E (eds) 1983 Stress reduction and prevention. Plenum Press, New York

Oakley-Brown M 1991 The epidemiology of anxiety disorders. International Journal of Psychiatry 3:243–252

Ost L G, Breitholtz E 2000 Applied relaxation vs cognitive therapy in the treatment of generalised anxiety disorder. Behaviour Research and Therapy 38:777–790

Rasmussen S A, Tsuang, M T 1986 Clinical characteristics and family history in DSM-III obsessive compulsive disorder. American Journal of Psychiatry 1943:317–382

Reich J H 1986 The epidemiology of anxiety. Journal of Nervous and Mental Disease 174:129–136

Reich J, Noyes R, Troughton E 1987 Dependent personality disorder associated with phobic avoidance in patients with panic disorder. American Journal of Psychiatry 144:323–326

Sanderson W C, DiNardo P A, Rapee R M et al 1990 Syndrome comorbidity in patients diagnosed with a DSM III-R anxiety disorder. Journal of Abnormal Psychology 99:308–312

Wells A 1997 Cognitive therapy of anxiety disorders: a practice manual and conceptual guide: Wiley, Chichester

Wells J E, Bushnell J A, Hornblow et al 1989 Christchurch psychiatric epidemiology study: methodology and lifetime prevalence for specific psychiatric disorders. Australian and New Zealand Journal of Psychiatry 23:315–326

Wolpe J 1958 Psychotherapy by reciprocal inhibition. Stanford University Press, Stanford, CA

Young J, Klosko J S, Weishaar M E 2003 Schema therapy: a practitioner's guide. Guilford, New York

Cognitive–Behavioural Interventions in Physiotherapy and Occupational Therapy

Enduring mental illness

Edward A S Duncan

6

Introduction

Enduring mental illness is an umbrella term for several conditions that have a long-term effect on individuals' lives. It is estimated that approximately 15,000 people in England experience enduring mental illness each year (Department of Health 1999). Frequently such individuals are supported and assisted by allied health professionals. This chapter reviews the contribution of a cognitive–behavioural perspective in the rehabilitation of individuals with enduring mental illness. The chapter commences with an overview of enduring mental illness, defining what it means and examining its effects. The chapter then continues by examining a variety of cognitive – behavioural therapy (CBT) interventions with enduring mental illness, before concluding with an overview of occupational therapy and physiotherapy for enduring mental illness.

What is enduring mental illness?

Typically, individuals with enduring mental illness have a psychotic or long-term depressive illness. A significant minority may have primary diagnoses of personality disorder or an organic disorder such as dementia, or drug or alcohol abuse, but these conditions are not directly considered within this chapter. Despite biological developments in the understanding and treatment of enduring mental illnesses, pharmacological approaches to intervention with this population often remain ineffective (Slade & Haddock 1996). CBT has a significant history of working with enduring mental illness. It was the focus of an early study by cognitive therapy's founding father Aaron Beck (Beck 1952) and was later embodied in his work on depression (Beck et al 1979). The intervening years have witnessed a hiatus in developments of CBT interventions for people with psychosis, as it was generally assumed that people with psychotic illnesses did not have the capacity to meaningfully engage in a didactic therapeutic relationship. However, since the 1990s there has been a developing evidence base for CBT interventions with people with psychosis. This work has predominantly emanated from the UK.

Key forms of CBT interventions for enduring mental illnesses have included interventions developed to address specific symptoms (Beck et al 1979; Bentall 1994; Chadwick & Birchwood 1994), interventions directed at enhancing individuals' coping skills (Tarrier et al 1990) and interventions that attempt to normalize the experience (Kingdon & Turkington 1991). Whilst these interventions are specifically designed CBT interventions, their key concepts offer much to support the work of occupational therapists and physiotherapists in practice and will be explored in greater depth within this chapter. Working with such individuals is characterized by complex long-term problems with individuals requiring support over a prolonged period of time. It is therefore important, for both client and therapist, that appropriate interventions are employed to assist clients obtain the highest achievable quality of life and functioning.

Definition

Various definitions of enduring mental illness exist. Kai et al (2000) define enduring mental illness as being equal to two or more years impaired social behaviour and inability to maintain any of the following roles: keeping a job, maintaining self-care, completing domestic chores, or taking part in recreational activities. Simmonds et al (2001, p 497) more broadly defines it as 'a psychiatric illness of sufficient severity to require intensive input and regular review'.

Characteristics of enduring mental illness

Characteristically people with enduring mental illness have a broad range of functional difficulties in their lives, with few areas unaffected. Morbidity and mortality is higher than average amongst individuals with enduring mental illness. This is not due in itself to the psychiatric components of enduring mental illness, but related issues, such as increased smoking, poor diet and lack of physical exercise that are frequently observed within this population (Phelan et al 2001).

Social functioning

Social functioning within this client group is frequently affected. This can result in restricted social networks and associated feelings of isolation and difficulties in relating to others. Difficulties in social functioning can be a vicious circle, with existing communication difficulties exacerbating and resulting in further isolation, which in turn leads to greater isolation. Another aspect of difficulties in social functioning can be a diminished sense of social awareness.

Cognitive functioning

Cognitive functioning is also frequently affected and people often present with diminished ability of emotional expression and decreased volition. A brief consideration of the profound effects that a diminished capacity in these areas of functioning would have on your own life illustrates the impact of enduring mental illness on everyday activity. A further illustration of the effects of enduring mental illness is presented in Case Study 6.1.

Historically, individuals with enduring mental illness were largely cared for in psychiatric institutions. The introduction of community care has, however, significantly impacted on the extent of inpatient care and length of patient stay. Whilst many negative comments could be made regarding the institutionalization of individuals with enduring mental illness, such environments did provide a true sense of asylum (or safety), where individuals' unusual behaviour was tolerated or understood. Integrating individuals with enduring mental illness within society offers many opportunities, but the sense of safety that frequently accompanied staying in a hospital setting can often be lost and ironically the community in which a person lives may not be so caring and can increase an individual's sense of isolation and fear.

CASE STUDY 6.1

Harry is a 54-year-old man, living on his own in a small flat. He was diagnosed with schizophrenia when he was 23 years old whilst serving in the armed forces and was discharged on medical grounds. At this time, Harry's fiancée separated from him and he spent several months resident in his local psychiatric hospital. Harry then lived with his parents, who provided his main care for several years. Both parents died several years ago. Although Harry has had some brief periods of employment since leaving the army, he has not worked for the last 15 years. Harry's motivation is very low and he often does not get out of bed until the early afternoon. His self-care is also poor and his dietary intake is very poor. Harry does receive regular input from members of his community mental health team (CMHT), including his occupational therapist and his community psychiatric nurse. The CMHT have arranged a variety of activities for Harry including an exercise class for people with enduring mental illness which is run by a physiotherapist who provides sessions input to the CMHT. Other than the arranged input, Harry largely spends his time in his kitchen smoking. He has no visitors and finds it difficult to relate to people.

CBT and enduring mental illness

A normalizing approach

Working with individuals with enduring mental illness, particularly those who have a psychotic condition, can initially be unnerving. Such people will undergo a wide range of unusual experiences (e.g. auditory, visual, tactile or olfactory hallucinations). Historically, therapists were encouraged to ignore such experiences, as to discuss them may exacerbate a person's condition or would prove a fruitless venture (Scharfetter 1980). Whilst such a position is not supported by the existing evidence base, it remains a prevalent belief amongst a wide range of health-care practitioners. More recently, research (Kingdon & Turkington 1991) has demonstrated that active engagement, collaboration and normalization of psychotic experiences decreases individuals' rates of readmission to psychiatric hospitals and reduces levels of suicide.

Developing a meaningful relationship with people who experience enduring mental illness

Developing a meaningful therapeutic relationship with individuals who experience enduring mental illness is vital to ensure therapeutic success. Turkington & Kingdon (1996) outline several key features of engaging with people with enduring mental illness and building rapport. These features are relevant regardless of the client's diagnosis; however, examples are given in the following sections that relate to specific diagnosis to illustrate certain issues.

Empathy and warmth

All the features of a collaborative therapeutic relationship, including empathy, warmth and understanding are equally valid when working with people with enduring mental illness.

Most clinicians agree it is important to be empathic. To a certain extent empathy is viewed as a therapeutic essential. The danger of this, however, is that the art of therapeutic empathy can be reduced to a basic communication skill. Instead, empathy is a complex communication skill in which a person listens and attends to all that is – and is not – said. Therapeutic empathy is an active process, one which Gilbert refers to as being in tune with the client (Gilbert 2007). It is also informative to consider what empathy is not. Empathy should not be confused with sympathy. Sympathy refers to a therapist's experience of wanting to alleviate pain and give reassurance. Conversely, empathy involves developing a deeper awareness of the person's experiences and communicating that you understand (at a profound level) what they are telling you. Finally it is important to convey warmth to a client. This helps them feel accepted, valued and within the therapeutic relationship.

Experience of working with people with enduring mental illness

Each individual with enduring mental illness is unique. A person may present with a wide range of clinical features that include depression, hallucinations, delusions, thought disorder etc. Experience of the wide range of clinical presentations over time will increase a therapist's confidence in working with such people.

Be consistent and respectful

Developing a therapeutic relationship with people who are, by the nature of their difficulties, inconsistent is very important and takes time. Confrontational responses to beliefs, including psychotically driven beliefs, may often damage a carefully developed relationship. Similarly, colluding with an individual and agreeing with beliefs that appear to be psychotically driven is unhelpful, both to a person's recovery and to your developing therapeutic relationship. The most effective response to challenging questions or statements from individuals with enduring mental illness is to tread the tightrope between confrontation and collaboration (Turkington & Kingdon 1996). For example, if a client was to declare that his house was being attacked with rays from aliens in space, an appropriate answer would be to acknowledge that it must be very distressing to have that belief, but highlight that from your perspective, such a possibility would be very remote, as no proof of aliens has yet been confirmed – despite significant research. A further step would be to collaborate with the client and suggest he find out further information about the possibility of this belief as part of his 'homework' for the next time you meet.

Despite such collaboration, clients will, on occasion, continue to firmly hold onto such beliefs. On these occasions continued persuasion (even if collaborative and non-confrontational in nature) can distress a client. On such occasions, further attempts to rationalize with such individuals are counterproductive and it is more helpful to acknowledge that people can agree to differ (Turkington & Kingdon 1996).

Feeling comfortable when working with actively ill individuals

Staying beside an individual who is actively unwell and delivering seemingly unclear and disjointed conversation can be, at least initially, very offputting. Developing this skill has been likened to allowing 'waves of psychosis to roll over you' (Turkington & Kingdon 1996, p 105). Such a skill is crucial for building a useful therapeutic relationship in this context. As a therapist gets to know a client, seemingly disjointed statements can often be more clearly understood in light of that person's personal history and development.

Educating an individual in the cognitive model of enduring mental illness

Unlike traditional CBT, the therapeutic process of working with people with enduring mental illness should be expected to take place over a considerably longer period of time and in shorter bursts, due to reduced concentration span. The essential components of the CBT process (see Chapter 1) remain the same.

Explaining symptoms

Experiencing psychotic symptoms is very distressing. Frequently, people may become aware of their diagnosis from a family member, realize themselves, or recognize their experiences from media portrayals. The realization of being seriously mentally ill is an anxiety-provoking experience and individuals will frequently develop unhelpful beliefs such as, 'I am going mad' or 'I will be locked up forever'. Such experiences, in turn, may increase an individual's frequency and intensity of symptomatology and lead to increased distress. It is often useful to educate individuals about the stress vulnerability model (Zubin & Spring 1977) in which increase of stress, or exposure to stressful conditions is known to lead to the increased potential to experience psychotic symptoms. It can also be useful to discuss the range of potential factors that are known to lead to a person experiencing distressing psychotic symptoms. Such factors include:

- Sleep deprivation
- Post-traumatic stress disorder
- Sensory deprivation
- Being taken hostage
- Isolation or solitary confinement
- Sexual abuse (Turkington & Kingdon 1996).

95

The knowledge that psychotic symptoms are experienced by a far wider group of people than many initially realize can be both reassuring and destigmatizing for the individuals concerned.

Coping strategy enhancement

Coping strategy enhancement (CSE) is a very pragmatic approach to working with people who have an enduring mental illness. The focus of this approach is on symptom maintenance (Yusupoff & Tarrier 1996). Within CSE, positive psychotic symptoms, such as hallucinations and delusions, are viewed as occurring within a social and emotional context. Furthermore, psychotic symptoms are seen as being unlikely to exist outwith such contexts and are likely to be affected by them. Within a CSE approach, the first significant step is to gain a detailed reaction of how the client emotionally responds when the symptoms are present. Such information can be used, in collaboration with the client, throughout traditional cognitive–behavioural therapy techniques, part of which is to test reality. Existing coping strategies may not be helpful, or may appear to be effective but in practice serve to maintain clients' symptoms and avoid difficulties (Yusupoff & Tarrier 1996). In acknowledging the importance of contextual material, CSE does not suggest that background factors cause psychotic episodes, rather that it can be helpful to the therapeutic process to acknowledge the influence that contextual factors and individuals psychological processes can have on clients.

Motivation is another key factor which is considered within CSE. Whilst experiencing an enduring mental illness is understandably viewed as a negative experience, it is true that such experiences can also be viewed positively. Miller et al (1993) reported that 53% of clients found their hallucinations in some way helpful (e.g. they were relaxing, or kept the client company). Unsurprisingly, therefore, clients' perspectives of improving may vary according to their attitudes to the cost of such an improvement in their life (e.g. a client with an ongoing psychotic illness may be reluctant to get better as they would then 'miss the voices for company' or may be fearful that an increase in their well-being could be accompanied by a decrease in their support).

Coping strategy enhancement interventions

Within a CSE framework, considerable variation of interventions can be used, depending upon the desired goal and the nature of the psychotic stimuli (hallucinations, delusions, or both). A comprehensive assessment is vital and standardized assessments (such as the Present State Examination (Wing et al 1974)) are often used to support this process. Having established the nature of the psychotic phenomena experienced by the client, a cognitive–behavioural analysis of each symptom is then undertaken. This process enables greater information to be gathered about the specific contexts, emotional reactions and symptom beliefs that a client holds about their experiences. This process also enables the therapist to understand the helpful and unhelpful coping strategies that a client is currently using to cope with their psychotic experiences (Yusupoff & Tarrier 1996). Coping strategies that support the reduction of stress from psychotic experiences and do not result in avoidance behaviour are supported and strategies that are unhelpful are discouraged.

Symptom generation can also be used to recreate the emotional reactions that a client can experience together with their psychotic experiences. Such an approach is not always possible, however, and guided imagery can also be used for a similar purpose. Having elicited the client's emotional reactions, it is possible to access their 'hot cognitions' (Duncan 2006) and the thoughts and feelings that accompany the experiences, thus opening the potential for more traditional CBT interventions.

Activity scheduling

Individuals with enduring mental illness frequently display difficulties in motivating themselves to initiate or complete activities. Activity scheduling is the process through which both therapist and clients agree on a programme of activities that the client will undertake, usually set, and reviewed, on a weekly basis. It is an intervention that is well known to occupational therapists, physiotherapists and cognitive–behavioural therapists (Duncan 2003). The development of an activity schedule can often be important in supporting the collaborative relationship between a therapist and client. Important issues to consider when setting up an activity schedule with a client who has enduring mental illness are:

- Ensure that the activities selected are meaningful to the client.
- Do not overload the timetable – it is better to start small and have successes than to aim high and not manage.

In their seminal work on cognitive therapy for depression, Beck et al (1979) highlight that developing an effective activity schedule with clients may 'tax the therapist's ingenuity to get the patient sufficiently involved in the idea of carrying out a program of activities or even filling in his activity schedule retrospectively' (p 121). Beck et al (1979) make several suggestions that can assist in making activity scheduling an effective intervention:

- Explain the rationale behind activity scheduling and emphasize that the first goal is to follow the schedule rather than feel 'better'. Improved health will follow improved functioning.
- Discover if the client has any objections to developing and using an activity schedule.
- If clients do object or are sceptical then suggest to use it as an experiment and see what effect it has.

Beck et al (1979) go on to emphasize that clients should not expect themselves to achieve everything on their schedule, activities should state what they will do, not *how much* they will achieve: this can be dependent on a range of factors, and is often beyond the control of the client. Trying to accomplish the activities listed in the schedule should be viewed as a success in itself. If the client is unable to achieve all they set out to then it may be a sign that the goals were too high and the schedule should be revised to incorporate more achievable activities. Making the activity schedule a part of a client's routine is essential to its success. Clients should be encouraged to regularly review and complete the schedule. An example of an activity schedule for Ania is illustrated in Table 6.1.

Table 6.1 ● First stages of graded activity skill development programme

	Monday	**Tuesday**	**Wednesday**	**Thursday**	**Friday**	**Saturday**	**Sunday**
AM		Go to local shop for groceries		Clean flat			
PM	Go for short walk in local park (weather permitting)		Go to exercise class		Attend community group in library		
EVE							

Skills training

We all need a variety of skills to meaningfully and productively participate in daily life: skills to survive, e.g. preparing and eating food; skills to be a part of the community, e.g. social skills; mastery of public transport; and skills to develop our personal identity, e.g. in work and leisure (Roberts 2002). Enduring mental illness can have a profound effect on an individual's abilities to use their everyday skills, which often deteriorate significantly over a period of time. Skills training frequently takes the form of behavioural therapy (Bellack et al 1997).

Skill deficits in people with enduring mental illness can be attributable to both acute 'positive' symptoms and 'negative' symptoms associated with the ongoing nature of the illness. Skill deficit can relate to difficulty completing tasks due to hallucinatory experiences or paranoid beliefs such as a belief that the washing machine is watching you or due to negative symptoms that emerge over time and can erode individuals' volition and sense of personal worth, therefore making self-care activities more challenging and apparently less important. Similarly skills training can also frequently be helpful for people with depression. Individuals with affective disorders experience skills deficits; these can develop from self-confidence being undermined and a loss of confidence in a person's own worth. A vicious cycle can often be seen to emerge, where an individual's confidence and sense of self-worth decreases, leading to situations of avoidance. Consequently, individuals have fewer opportunities to sustain their social and life-skill developments and therefore avoid social situations. This in turn leads to further loss of confidence and self-worth and the difficulties continue in a vicious circle, as illustrated in Case Study 6.2.

CASE STUDY 6.2

Ania is a 42-year-old Polish woman. Two years ago she emigrated to Scotland from her native Poland with her husband and two children. Ania describes experiencing postnatal depression after the birth of her second child (a girl) six years ago. She recovered gradually from this experience but states her self-confidence has never returned to the level it was at prior to the birth of her daughter. Before having her first child Ania was an office administrator in a large factory in Krakow. She left this post to look after her children. Since arriving in Scotland, Ania has felt that her depression is increasing once more. Her husband works in a local factory and is away from the house most days. Both her children attend their local primary school. Ania states she has little social contact other than with a few Polish women, whom she now rarely arranges to meet. She presented herself to her GP and described low mood, lethargy, sleep disturbance and a lack of confidence in completing everyday tasks such as shopping. After initially prescribing an antidepressant, without significant success, the GP referred Ania to a primary care mental health team where she was allocated to an occupational therapist.

Following an initial assessment, Ania stated that she felt she was lacking in the confidence to complete tasks that she previously undertook, such as shopping and using the phone. Together, Ania and the occupational therapists agreed to develop a plan to help Ania re-establish her skills in shopping, planning what to buy, selecting items, and paying for and packing her goods and to increase her confidence and mastery in completing her shopping and using the phone. Initially the occupational therapist role-played shopping scenarios with Ania and a graded activity programme was then established to assist Ania in skill development (see Table 6.1).

Key stages of engagement

Assessment

A variety of assessments exist which merit consideration when working with people who have an enduring mental illness, including a range of cognitive–behavioural measures. Some occupational therapy assessments may also be helpful. Both CBT and occupational therapy assessments generally fall into the following categories: checklists; structured and semi-structured interviews; third party reports (e.g. carers); and observations.

Careful consideration should be given to the use of client-led forms of assessment as such individuals may have difficulties in concentration and assessments that rely on client completion of checklists or interviews may prove excessively burdensome. That said, it is vital that the client is involved in any assessment procedure. Therefore, shorter, but more frequent periods of contact with a client should be considered when gathering information. Carers can often provide a valuable perspective of what a client's needs and abilities are. However, observation of an individual over a period of time and on separate occasions is perhaps the most complete method of assessment.

General assessments

Several general assessments can be of use when working with people who have an enduring mental illness. These assessments, are general screening assessments, and can be of particular use when a client is met for the first time. These assessments include the following.

The General Health Questionnaire (GHQ) (Goldberg & Williams 1988) This questionnaire focuses on two major aspects of health – an inability to carry out normal functions and the appearance of new and distressing phenomena. Three versions of the GHQ exist: the GHQ-60: the fully detailed 60-item questionnaire; the GHQ-30: a short form without items relating to physical illness (not so relevant for the population under consideration); the GHQ-28: a 28-item scaled version which assesses somatic symptoms, anxiety and insomnia, social dysfunction and severe depression; and the GHQ-12: a quick, reliable and sensitive short form often used in research studies.

The Symptom Checklist-90-R (SCL-90-R) (Derogatis et al 1973) The SCL-90-R evaluates a wide range of psychological problems and symptoms. It can also be helpful in measuring clients' progress and treatment outcomes. Its use is both clinical and research and can be used by a wide range of health professionals. The SCL-90-R has been found to be helpful when:

- Initially evaluating clients as an objective method for symptom screening
- Evaluating client progress during and after intervention
- As a part of an interventions outcome measurement
- In research to assist in the measurement of symptom shift.

Occupational therapy specific assessments

A variety of occupational therapy specific measures exist. The Model of Human Occupation Screening Tool (MOHOST) (Parkinson et al 2006), is a relatively new occupational therapy assessment that was specifically designed for individuals with lower levels of functioning and volition, such as individuals with enduring mental illnesses. The MOHOST was developed in line with the Model of Human Occupation (MOHO) (Kielhofner 2002), a well-known and frequently used conceptual model of practice in occupational therapy (see Chapter 2 for a fuller discussion). The Model of Human Occupation is fundamentally an occupation-focused understanding of human beings. It provides the theoretical understanding and practical instruments, such as assessments, to assist occupational therapists to undertake their professional role and responsibility. The MOHO, however, does not provide any 'theory of mind' and it is here that CBT has significant contributions to make (Duncan 2006). The MOHOST is structured in the form of five sections (motivation for occupation, pattern for occupation, communication and interaction, process skills and motor skills), with four separate factors in each section. Each factor is rated on a rating scale from 1 (Deficient) to 4 (Competent). The MOHOST is a good example of an occupational therapy specific assessment that gathers robust information that can assist in the prioritization and formulation of an intervention plan. Other occupational therapy measures exist and may also be beneficial in gathering information and as a baseline and future outcome measure.

Cognitive–behavioural assessments

Cognitive–behavioural measures can also be used. Specific assessments for individuals with enduring mental illness exist. These include the Psychotic Symptoms Rating Scale, which has two subscales: the auditory hallucinations scale and the delusions scale (Haddock et al 1999). This measure comprehensively assesses the nature and degree of psychotic stimuli experienced by a client. These measures can also be used as outcome measures to observe changes in levels of psychotic stimuli as intervention continues. Further information about specific CBT scales can be found in more specialist texts, for example Greenberger & Padesky (1995) include several measures for depression, and Haddock & Slade (1995) include an overview of several measures for psychotic disorders.

Intervention

Two potential manners of using CBT as a form of intervention have been presented:

- As a specific form of psychological intervention; or
- Integrated within the core role of the professional (i.e. as a component part of a person's occupational therapy or physiotherapy).

Several books exist that discuss intervention methods for the former mode of psychological intervention and outlines of specific interventions have been given within this chapter. This chapter focuses on the latter, i.e. as a part of the professional's core role in therapy.

Whilst physiotherapists and occupational therapists could gain further specialist training in CBT, and some do, many people choose not to, or are unable to undertake such training, but do desire to incorporate the principles of CBT into their practice. This can be achieved in several ways. For example, the maintenance of a supportive and collaborative therapeutic relationship, using a normalizing approach, would be a useful strategy for a physiotherapist to employ when working with an adult with psychosis attending a physiotherapy outpatient appointment. Within occupational therapy, the clinician may develop an activity schedule, in collaboration with a client who is experiencing from depression. Both of these activities would be regarded as 'core' to the profession's practice and both can be supported through the appropriate use of cognitive–behavioural theory and technique.

Conclusion

Occupational therapists and physiotherapists will come across people with enduring mental illness in the course of their professional practice; frequently in mental health settings, less frequently – but still occurring – in physical health settings. This chapter has presented an overview of the problems that people with enduring mental illness experience and outlined various differing strategies that CBT offers for working with and assisting people who have an enduring mental illness. The nature of this chapter entails that only an overview of several differing strategies can be given. More information and potentially supervision should be sought by any practitioner who wishes to directly employ these strategies in clinical practice.

 Key Messages

- Enduring mental illness constitutes a significant part of the workload of the mental health team.
- CBT provides a useful framework for assessment and treatment with this population.
- Occupational therapists and physiotherapists require well-developed interpersonal skills to facilitate communication with this patient/client group.
- CBT is effective in the management of positive and negative symptoms associated with psychotic conditions.

References

Beck A 1952 Successful out-patient psycho-therapy of a chronic schizophrenic with a delusion based on borrowed guilt. Psychiatry 15:305–312

Beck A, Rush A J, Shaw B F et al 1979 Cognitive therapy for depression. Guilford, New York

Bellack A S, Mueser K T, Gingerich S et al 1997 Social skills training for schizophrenia. Guilford, New York

Bentall R P 1994 Cognitive biases and abnormal beliefs: towards a model of persecutory delusions. In: David A S, Cutting J (eds) The neuropsychology of schizophrenia. Lawrence Erlbaum Associates, London

Chadwick P, Birchwood M 1994 Challenging the omnipotence of voices. British Journal of Psychiatry 164:190–201

Department of Health 1999 National service framework for mental health. DoH, London

Derogatis L R, Lipman R S, Covi L 1973 SCL-90: An outpatient psychiatric rating scale – preliminary report. Psychopharmacology Bulletin 9:13–17

Duncan E A S 2003 Cognitive-behavioural therapy in physiotherapy and occupational therapy. In: Everett T, Donaghy M, Feaver S (eds) Interventions for mental health: an evidence based approach. Butterworth Heinemann

Duncan E A S 2006 The cognitive-behavioural frame of reference. In: Duncan E A S (ed) Foundations for Practice in Occupational Therapy, 4th edn. Elsevier/Churchill Livingstone, Edinburgh, pp 217–232

Gilbert P 2007 Counselling for depression, 3rd edn. Sage, London

Goldberg D, Williams P 1988 A user's guide to the general health questionnaire. NFER-Nelson, Windsor

Greenberger D, Padesky C A 1995 Mind over mood: change how you feel by changing the way you think. Guilford, New York

Haddock G, Slade P D (eds) 1995 Cognitive-behavioural Interventions with psychotic disorders. Routledge, London

Haddock G, McCarron J, Tarrier N et al 1999 Scales to measure dimensions of hallucinations and delusions: the psychotic symptom rating scales (PSYRATS). Psychological Medicine 29(4):879–889

Kai J, Crosland A, Drinkwater C 2000 Prevalence of enduring and disabling mental illness in the inner city. British Journal of General Practice 50:988–994

Kielhofner G 2002 A model of human occupation: theory and application, 3rd edn. Williams and Wilkins, Baltimore

Kingdon D G, Turkington D 1991 The use of cognitive-behaviour therapy with a normalising rational in schizophrenia. Journal of Nervous and Mental Disease 179:207–211

Miller L J, O'Conner E, DiPasquale T 1993 Patients attitudes toward hallucinations. American Journal of Psychiatry 150:584–588

Parkinson S, Forsyth K, Kielhofner G 2006 The model of human occupation (V2). MOHO Clearing House

Phelan M, Stradins L, Morrison S 2001 Physical health of people with severe mental illness. British Medical Journal 322:443–444

Roberts M 2002 Life and social skills training. In: Creek J (ed) Occupational therapy in mental health. Churchill Livingstone, Edinburgh

Scharfetter C 1980 General psychopathology (translated H Marshall). Cambridge University Press, Cambridge

Simmonds S, Coid J, Joseph P, Marriott S, Tyrer P 2001 Community mental health team management in severe mental illness: a systematic review. British Journal of Psychiatry 178:487–502

Slade P D, Haddock G 1996 Historical overview of psychological treatment for psychotic symptoms. In: Haddock G, Slade P (eds) Cognitive-behavioural interventions with psychotic disorders. Routledge, London, pp 28–44

Tarrier N, Harwood S, Yusopoff L et al 1990 Coping strategy enhancement (CSE): a method of treating residual schizophrenic symptoms. Behavioural Psychotherapy 18:283–293

Turkington D, Kingdon D C 1996 Using a normalizing rational in the treatment of schizophrenic patients: In: Haddock G, Slade P (eds) Cognitive-behavioural interventions with psychotic disorders. Routledge, London

Wing J K, Cooper J E, Sartorious N 1974 Measurement and classification of psychiatric symptoms. Cambridge University Press, Cambridge

Yusupoff L, Tarrier N 1996 Coping strategy enhancement for persistent hallucinations and delusions. In: Haddock G, Slade P (eds) Cognitive-behavioural interventions with psychotic disorders. Routledge, London, pp 86–102

Zubin J, Spring B 1977 Vulnerability – a new view of schizophrenia. Journal of Abnormal Psychology 86(2):103–124

Cognitive–behavioural approaches in the treatment of alcohol addiction

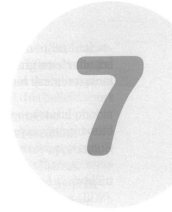

Marie Donaghy

Introduction

Addiction to alcohol is a global public health problem (World Health Organization 2004) with alcohol use and abuse by children and adolescents highlighted as a critical problem for modern developed countries (Bukstein & Trunzo 2005). The focus of this chapter is to provide a summary of risk and those most at risk, to look at the evidence for cognitive–behavioural therapy (CBT) in alcohol rehabilitation and to discuss the usefulness of CBT approaches illustrated by a case study.

Prevalence

The general household survey (Office of National Statistics 2005a) indicates that the heaviest drinkers are in the age group 16–24, with 47% of men and 39% of women exceeding the guidelines on one or more days of the week. The 16–24 age group is also more likely to engage in binge drinking, with 32% of men and 24% of women drinking more than 8 units in one day. The rise in women engaging in binge drinking has risen by 2% in two years. Alcohol use in adolescents is also increasing across Europe with a 2% increase in the last 10 years. The Nordic countries, UK, Ireland, Slovenia and Latvia have the highest levels of drunkenness with binge drinking reported at least three times in the last month by 31% of boys and 33% of girls between the ages of 15 and 16 (Hibell et al 2004). Across the whole of the EU, 1 in 8 (13%) of 15–16-year-olds have been drunk more than 20 times in their life and over 1 in 6 (18%) have binged five or more drinks on a single occasion (Hibell et al 2004). The reasons why young people drink vary; in the UK, 12–13-year-olds have indicated that they drink to signal the change from child to adult, while 14–15-year-olds indicate that getting drunk both tests their own ability to consume alcohol in large quantities but also to socialize (Honess et al 2000). Coleman & Cater (2005) found that where adolescents were seeking a 'buzz' from intoxication, rather than using alcohol for social facilitation, outcomes were found to be more harmful. Alcohol use in pre-adolescents and adolescents may be confounded with other addictions such as eating disorders. Conason & Sher's (2006) school-based studies highlight that amongst bulimics and binge eaters those that use alcohol and other drugs are more likely to engage in high-risk behaviours such as stealing and unprotected sex and are more likely to attempt suicide than restricting anorexics.

Morbidity

The World Health Organization's (WHO) comparative risk assessment study describes the relationship between alcohol consumption and health and social outcomes as complex and multi-dimensional (Rehm et al 2004), suggesting that the impact of alcohol on health occurs through three intermediate and linked variables; direct biochemical effects, intoxication and episodic heavy drinking and dependence (Figure 7.1). Those who are dependent on alcohol have an increased risk of developing up to 60 different types of diseases and conditions including chronic liver disease, cancer of the larynx and oesophagus, cerebrovascular disease, type 2 diabetes, injuries through accidents, increased depression and anxiety and low self-esteem (Anderson & Baumberg 2006). Damage to the musculoskeletal system from alcohol abuse is linked to poor physical fitness, skeletal muscle damage and loss of bone mass (Donaghy & Mutrie 1999). Alcohol is the third leading risk factor for death and disability in the EU, nearly four times that of illicit drugs; only blood pressure and smoking account for greater morbidity risk. In the UK provision of medical and social services for problem drinkers runs into billions of pounds, accounting for as much 12% of total NHS expenditure on hospitals in the UK (Royal College

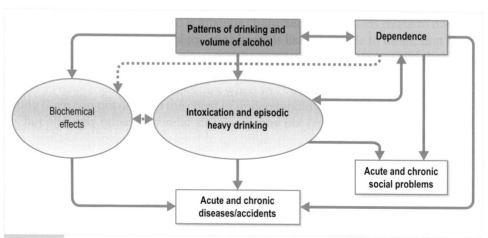

Figure 7.1 • The relationship between alcohol consumption, health and social outcomes (adapted from Rehm et al 2004).

of Physicians 2001). Treating associated illness in the EU costs 17 billion euros a year with an additional 5 billion euros spent on alcohol rehabilitation treatment (Rehm et al 2004).

Mortality

Among problem drinkers, chronic liver disease is the major cause of death. Mexico and the USA have the highest mortality rates from alcoholic liver disease per capita with 13,581 and 12,109 deaths, Japan the sixth highest with 3151 deaths, Canada lies in tenth place with 1104 deaths and the UK 14th with 866 deaths per million (Nationmaster 2004). Of the current 25 EU countries, deaths from alcohol account for 195,000 deaths per year and are responsible for 4.5 million disability adjusted life years, every year (Anderson & Baumberg 2006). In the UK alone in 2004, alcohol abuse was responsible for the death of 5465 males and 2915 females (Office of National Statistics 2005b). This is a 100% increase in the last 15 years. While the highest increase in mortality is in the 35–54 age group (105% in females and 150% in males), the increase in the 15–34 age group (33% in females and 75% in males) highlights the growing link between early onset drinking and mortality (Office of National Statistics 2005b).

Defining addiction

The WHO (2005) defines addiction as the repeated use of a psychoactive substance or substances to the extent that the user is periodically or chronically intoxicated, shows a compulsion to take the preferred substance, has great difficulty in modifying substance use and exhibits determination to obtain psychoactive substances by almost any means. Problem drinkers often consume well in excess of 50 units a week for males and 35 units a week for females. They are usually unable to stop for long periods of time and usually suffer withdrawal phenomena such as nausea, vomiting, tremors and shaking when the individual stops drinking (American Psychiatric Association 1994).

Cognitive–behavioural approach to treatment

The principles of Bandura's (1986, 1997) social learning theory informs the cognitive–behavioural approach to treatment. This approach assumes that addictive behaviours, including alcohol, are learned maladaptive habitual patterns acquired through the interactive processes of classical and operant conditioning and cognitive mediation. The cognitive–behavioural approach emphasizes to clients that excessive drinking is something they do, is not a disease, and that they have the ability to change their excessive drinking behaviour. By taking an active role in the planning and decision making throughout treatment there is a progressive shift in personal responsibility, with the aim being that the client becomes their own therapist over time as they gain new knowledge and skills with self-management being the ultimate treatment outcome.

Coping and social skills training are the core elements of cognitive–behavioural approaches for treating alcohol problems. Cognitive coping skills include strategies that enable the individual to recognize cues and to take appropriate action to cope with psycho-physiological or cognitive reactions associated with urges or cravings to consume alcohol. Coping skills are aimed at increasing self-efficacy in order to remain abstinent from alcohol in high-risk situations. Interpersonal skills include techniques to increase positive social interactions and self-confidence minimizing negative social interactions and avoidance of others (O'Leary & Monti 2002). Self-efficacy develops by repeating and practising these skills and has been found to be an important variable in treatment planning and delivery (Long et al 2000).

Recovery from addiction requires commitment to change behaviour. Orford (1985) explains dependence as the confrontation between an awareness of the adverse consequences of the addictive behaviour and the desire to continue with an overlearned behaviour which is enjoyed, valued and relied upon. This implies that motivation to change behaviour is not a static decision but a constant battle between the perceived costs and benefits of the behaviour. Within this model the cycle of relapse and return to drinking can be seen as something that may occur time and time again (Kassel et al 1999). The five stages in the process of behavioural change, as described by Prochaska & Diclemente (1992), highlight the different cognitive processes involved at each stage (Figure 7.2). The process, while indicated sequentially, is not dependent on achieving each stage; relapse can occur at any stage in the cycle.

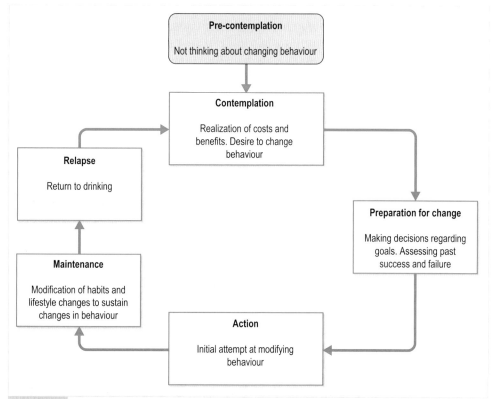

Figure 7.2 ● Stages of change (after Prochaska & Diclemente 1992).

Stages of change

The model of stages of change coupled with the explanation of addiction as described by Orford (1985) enables cognitive–behavioural strategies to be appropriately planned for the different stages. It will therefore be beneficial to know which stage the problem drinker is at when intervention is being considered. Saunders & Allsop (1991) suggest that intervention should be planned in four stages: resolution, commitment, action and maintenance.

Precontemplation

The precontemplation stage is unlikely to apply to anyone coming for treatment as that stage indicates satisfaction with their behaviour.

Contemplation – resolution

The first stage of intervention focuses on the decision that change is felt to be necessary. Motivational interviewing (Miller 1983) has been used as a strategy to encourage a cognitive self-appraisal of problems and concerns of recent drinking behaviour. It is seen as important that the problem drinker has carefully considered why they want to change their drinking behaviour (Miller & Rollnick 1991). A distinct form of counselling developed by Miller (1983) has been used to enhance individuals' resolve by helping them to face the realities of the situation and allowing them to decide what they wish their future behaviour to be. For a full explanation and description of the application of motivational interviewing see Rollnick & Allison (2001).

Preparation for change – commitment

The stage of commitment requires the problem drinker to participate in the planning of short- and long-term goals, with regard to their desired outcome. Whether that is abstinence or controlled drinking, at this planning stage it is important to give guidance on a range of behaviours and coping strategies that can build confidence. The importance of self-efficacy has been repeatedly demonstrated as a prognostic factor of change (Annis 1986). However, overconfidence may be present due to cognitive impairment with an unrealistic optimism about the ability to change behaviour (Saunders 1994). This preparation for change stage is seen as important with regard to firming up the commitment to change. Not infrequently, problem drinkers may take up treatment without having thought carefully about the commitment and the difficulties that they will face (Saunders 1994).

Action

In the action stage it has been shown that learning coping skills improves outcome of treatment (Heather & Tebbutt 1989). The range of skills useful for coping include relaxation skills, assertiveness training, stress management, problem-solving skill and relapse prevention – see Parks et al (2001) for a clinical guide to assessing and developing these skills. Donaghy & Ussher (2005) advocate exercise and increased physical activity to enhance self-esteem and lifestyle change as part of a planned coping strategy.

The use of cue exposure as a treatment to reduce the incidence of relapse has been frequently used. This work can be explained by considering 'impaired control' as a symptom that is central to addictive behaviour associated with problem drinking. To enable the problem drinker to improve their control, they are exposed to a powerful cue for further drinking. The exposure to a small number of drinks enables the problem drinker to practice resisting the urge to drink more. They learn that it is possible to regain control and resist the powerful cues by frequently repeating the behaviour (Saunders 1994). Conditioning theory underpins this work with the conditioned response in the above example being the desire to drink more which is gradually extinguished as control is learned. This practice can be linked to any powerful cue such as feelings of anxiety, particular environmental or situational cues etc. New knowledge on how to change implicit alcohol-related cognitions is also informing the field. In a recent study, problem drinkers were taught to use implementation intentions, for example a man who was experiencing anxiety who has previously been taught and rehearsed brief relaxation techniques to reduce the urge to drink in a situation in which he would previously have consumed alcohol (see also Chapter 1). Recent cognitive theories that integrate the role of attention with theories on how memories are processed and stored can also help us to understand the mechanisms involved in this procedure (Wiers et al 2006).

Maintenance

Social factors are also very important in the maintenance of change. Prochaska & Diclemente (1986) highlighted that social support such as the quality of familial support and opportunities for employment were vital in relation to the maintenance of change. These issues are critical to decisions with regard to contemplation and readiness to change. The presence of friends, close partner relationships, and group contact have all been found to be significantly associated with good outcome in giving up alcohol (Baucom et al 1998, Meyers & Smith 1997, Havassy et al 1991).

Relapse

Relapse from desired behaviour to familiar less desirable behaviour can be observed in all human behaviour. Relapse rates are high with 93% of clinic attendees found to return to problem drinking within four years (Polich et al 1980). The relapse model proposed by Marlatt & Gordon (1985) suggests that encounters with high-risk situations combined with a lack of successful coping are key reasons for the occurrence of relapse. There is evidence that problem drinkers display a cognitive processing bias that may contribute to relapse. One study comparing alcoholics and light drinkers demonstrated that alcoholics had enhanced memory recall for alcohol-related cues compared to other more neutral or general incentive cues; the magnitude of this bias in recall positively correlated with the magnitude of alcohol craving (Franken et al 2003).

Relapse should not be viewed as failure. The likelihood of relapse at some point and the action required to get back into the cycle of change at the appropriate stage has been clearly described by Marlatt & Gordon (1985). Some relapsers may move quickly back into the action stage (Trimpey 1989). The use of selective serotonin reuptake inhibitors (SSRIs), such as fluvoxamine, has been found to act as an adjunct to cognitive–behavioural therapy in reducing craving and maintaining abstinence (Angelone et al 1998) thus reducing likelihood of relapse.

Marlatt & Gordon's theory has been supported in a study of 122 attendees at an outpatient treatment clinic for alcohol problems (Miller et al 1996). Drinking status and a variety of predictor variables were measured every two months for one year following presentation for treatment. Potential antecedents included negative life events, cognitive appraisal variables including self-efficacy, alcohol expectancies, motivation for change, coping resources, craving experiences and affective/mood status. All variables with the exception of life events singly accounted for significant variance in drinking outcomes. Marlatt & Gordon's model was supported with two factors optimally predicting relapse – lack of coping skills and belief in the disease model of alcoholism (Miller et al 1996). Marlatt (1996) in a historical overview provided further evidence to support the clinical validity of the model and presented a refined and extended taxonomy of high-risk situations associated with his cognitive–behavioural model of relapse. This was followed by the Relapse Replication and Extension Project (Lowman et al 1996). This multisite study replicated and extended Marlatt's taxonomy of relapse precipitants.

The efficacy of cognitive therapy for alcohol addiction

In looking at the evidence to support the use of cognitive–behavioural therapy we need to explore the following: is it effective? Is it more effective than other treatments? Is there a causal link between theory and recovery?

Is it effective?

Evidence for the active ingredients of cognitive–behavioural therapy for patients with alcohol disorders was presented at the 2004 Research Society on Alcoholism conference in Vancouver (Longabaugh et al 2005). The evidence supporting the efficacy of this approach includes randomized controlled studies and meta-analysis. In a comprehensive review of alcohol treatment outcome studies, Miller & Hester (1995) suggest that the strongest evidence for cognitive–behavioural therapy in alcohol treatment is linked to social-skills training, community reinforcement approach, behavioural contracting, aversion therapy, cognitive therapy and relapse prevention. Long et al (2000) examining predictors of drinking outcome following cognitive–behavioural treatment highlights the importance of self-efficacy as a significant treatment variable in treatment planning and delivery.

Other studies have looked at the overall effectiveness of cognitive–behavioural approaches in relapse prevention and the extent to which certain variables may relate to treatment outcome. In a review by Irvin et al (1999), 26 published and unpublished studies representing a combined sample of 9,504 participants were included in a meta-analysis with the results indicating that relapse prevention is most effective when applied to alcohol- or polysubstance-use disorders, combined with the adjunctive use of medication such as fluvoxamine or naltrexone. Anton et al (1999) explored the effectiveness of cognitive–behavioural approaches when combined with naltrexone, an opiate antagonist, in a double-blind randomized clinical trial (RCT). The results of this well-controlled RCT suggests that when weekly outpatient CBT treatment is combined with naltrexone there is increased control over alcohol cravings and improved cognitive resistance to thoughts about drinking.

Not all effects of CBT are enhanced by naltrexone. Feeney et al (2004), in a study comparing the effectiveness of CBT against CBT with naltrexone, concluded that study participants who completed the CBT-only arm of the study reported significant improvements in self-report health status (SF-36) and well-being (GHQ-28); the adjunctive use of naltrexone did not improve these outcomes.

These findings are indicative that CBT is effective in developing coping strategies and that in relation to relapse prevention the effectiveness can be enhanced by using naltrexone or fluvoxamine (Angelone et al 1998) as an adjunct to therapy.

Is CBT more effective than other treatments?

The largest and most expensive study undertaken to compare cognitive–behavioural treatments (CBT) to the Twelve Step Alcoholics Anonymous Programme (TSP) and Motivational Enhancement Therapy (MET) is Project MATCH (Project MATCH post-treatment drinking outcomes, 1997). The aim of this study was to ascertain whether there were benefits in matching people with alcohol dependence to three different treatments with reference to a variety of client attributes. Two parallel but independent RCTs were conducted, one with people receiving outpatient treatment ($n = 952$; 72% male) and one where aftercare therapy was being received following inpatient or day hospital treatment ($n = 774$; 80% male). Study participants were randomly allocated to one of three 12-week, manual-guided, individually delivered treatments: cognitive coping-skills therapy, motivational enhancement therapy or 12-step facilitation therapy. Participants were monitored over a one-year post-treatment period. Primary outcome measures were days abstinent and alcoholic drinks per drinking day. Attendance was on average two-thirds of treatment sessions offered, and research follow-up rates exceeded 90% of living subjects interviewed at one year post-treatment. The results highlighted that there was no significant difference between the different treatment groups in terms of the primary outcomes. There was some evidence to suggest that study participants who were low in psychiatric severity had more abstinent days in the 12-step facilitation programme compared to those who had CBT. Other findings indicated that attributes such as motivational readiness, network for social support to avoid drinking alcohol, psychiatric severity and sociopathy were indicative of drinking outcomes over time, findings supported the existing literature. Further analysis concluded that in the outpatient arm 41% of CBT and TSP participants were abstinent or drank moderately compared to 28% of MET participants; these small but significant differences were not found in the other treatment arm (Project MATCH Matching alcoholism treatments to client heterogeneity 1998).

At three-year follow-up, the three treatment groups had similar outcomes in regard to abstinence levels and days drinking with 30% of the participants totally abstinent in months 37–39. Client traits did not prove to be prognostic factors; instead malleable states such as motivation, readiness to change, self-efficacy and social support were the strongest predictors of successful long-term drinking outcome (Miller & Longabaugh 2003).

In reviewing the findings of Project MATCH, which was the largest and most expensive alcoholism treatment trial ever conducted, Cutler & Fishbain (2005) concluded that there were essentially no patient–treatment matches and three very different treatment approaches produced nearly identical outcomes in regard to abstinence and drinks per drinking day. The results were interpreted and published as evidence that all three treatments were effective (Project MATCH 1997, 1998). To investigate this further, Cutler & Fishbain undertook secondary analysis of the data from the multisite clinical trial of alcohol-dependent volunteers ($n = 1726$) who received outpatient psychosocial therapy. Analysis of data was confined to the two primary outcomes, days abstinent and drinks per drinking day. Three groups were highlighted – those who dropped out prior to the start of treatment, those who dropped out after only one therapy session, and those who attended 12 therapy sessions. The results question the earlier claims of treatment efficacy. Findings suggest that a median of only 3% of the drinking outcome at follow-up can be attributed to treatment and that most of the improvement occurred within the first week of treatment. The authors conclude that current psychosocial treatments for alcohol treatment may not be particularly effective and that untreated alcoholics in clinical trials show significant improvement. These findings challenge the previously published claims from the MATCH project of efficacy of treatment and question the underpinning philosophies.

However, these findings should be interpreted with caution. Support for different approaches to treatment does not mean that all clients will benefit from these approaches, nor does it suggest that clients would not find some benefit from less effective approaches. There is also an established body of evidence indicating that alcoholics can overcome their dependence without extensive professional help (Klingemann & Gmel 2001) and that this process of self-change is usually triggered by social, financial or health problems. The design of the Project MATCH study may also have influenced outcome. A manualized approach was chosen to deliver the interventions; this combined with the careful monitoring of treatment sessions may have constrained the degree to which therapists could tailor treatment to the individual and may have made the approaches more similar than different.

At this time there is insufficient evidence to conclude that cognitive approaches to treatment are more effective than MET or TSP in relation to outcomes of number of drinking days or abstinence.

Is there a causal link between theory and recovery?

Morgenstern & Longabaugh (2000) reviewed 10 CBT studies which included randomization and comparative treatment groups to determine whether there was

113

a causal link between increased coping and recovery from alcohol addiction. The results failed to establish this link. While there is a substantive body of evidence supporting the inclusion of CBT as an effective treatment for alcohol dependence the causal link between coping and recovery has yet to be established. The findings of Cutler & Fishbain (2005) challenge the theoretical basis on which current psychosocial treatments have been based. Taking into account the complexities of addiction and its effects on health and behaviour (Figure 7.1) it is perhaps not surprising that to date we have not been able to establish a causal link between theory and recovery. It is more likely that the links between theory and recovery are multifaceted and interdependent, making it complex to determine. These links are likely to include cognitive, behavioural, social and biological explanations.

Exercise and cognitive–behavioural approaches

In a recent critical review of the literature, Donaghy & Ussher (2005) found some evidence to support the use of exercise as an adjunct in the treatment of alcohol and drug addiction. Their findings highlight unequivocal support that physical exercise regimens have a positive effect on aerobic fitness and strength if administered as an adjunct in alcohol rehabilitation. This may be important to people who want to change their lifestyle, engaging with social groups where a healthy lifestyle is the focus. Support for a positive effect on physical self-perceptions was found in one RCT, entailing a 3–4-week strength and aerobic exercise regimen within an alcohol rehabilitation programme; this was maintained by continuing in a 12-week home-based programme of exercise. There is also some evidence to support a link between improvements in self-esteem and exercise with alcohol and drug rehabilitation. These changes may be important in giving people confidence that they can attain their goals to change their behaviour. Experimental evidence from one study suggests that alcohol cravings may be alleviated during exercise; for some people this may assist in relapse prevention. While overall the evidence for exercise improving abstinence levels or controlled drinking levels is at this time equivocal, Donaghy (1997) emphasizes the importance of linking positive outcomes from exercise with coping strategies. As stated earlier, there are a number of strategies available to clients to assist in changing their drinking behaviour. Exercise can be used in conjunction with relaxation training or as an alternative approach to reduce the physiological symptoms of stress (Parks et al 2001) and to move towards a healthier lifestyle and a better quality of life. Exercise can be integrated into the preparation, action and maintenance stages of change. These are outlined in Case Study 7.1.

CASE STUDY 7.1

Angela Smith is a 34-year-old woman with a five-year history of problem drinking, attending an out-patient rehabilitation programme for the second time; her previous attempt 18 months ago resulted in relapse after 4 months of abstinence. Angela has also been a regular cannabis user with occasional use of ecstasy. Angela is a single mum with a 7-year-old son; she is currently unemployed and they live in a multistorey flat in an inner-city area of high social deprivation.

Assessment

The initial assessment brought together information from the client's medical history with that of recent drinking behaviour. The Brief Drinking Profile and the Timeline Follow-back Method (Donovan & Marlatt 1988, Sobell & Sobell 1993) were used to ascertain levels of alcohol dependence and the nature and severity of alcohol-related problems. It is important to establish the antecedents of drinking behaviour such as time, place, people, activities, the triggers and repeated behaviours that initiate it, the pattern of drinking itself including daily/weekly consumption and the consequences that reinforce the drinking. Angela's drinking started in the morning once her son went to school; she drank alone watching TV, consequently feeling relaxed and more confident. She had very few friends; a number of the other single mums living close to her were regular heroin users and she was afraid that if she socialized with them she would be drawn into more regular illicit drug use. The importance of self-monitoring of drinking behaviour, the keeping of a diary and undertaking homework between sessions was discussed and agreed.

Motivational interview

In order to establish Angela's commitment to changing her drinking behaviour motivational interviewing techniques were employed. Rollnick & Allison (2001) describe motivational interviewing as a counselling style that facilitates an atmosphere of constructive conversation in which the health professional uses empathetic listening to gain insight into the client's perspective of their drinking behaviour and what they would like to change. During this interview it became evident that Angela had reservations about changing her behaviour. While she recognized that her excessive drinking was linked to low mood and was affecting her ability to function normally, she still saw drinking as being her only way to deal with feelings of stress. The recognition of other health-associated problems and the exploration of potential desired end points and goals were explored. One of her goals was to get back to feeling fit again. Prior to having her son, Angela had attended aerobic exercise classes. However, at this point there were a number of barriers that prevented her from seeing how she could do this, including: feeling self-conscious about her appearance, low levels of confidence regarding ability to undertake an aerobic class, and low self-esteem.

Strategies

Over the next three sessions a number of strategies were explored to cope with cravings for alcohol and urges to drink. Angela kept a diary, noting key triggers that stimulated the desire to drink; this included mood and strength of craving as well as external cues such as observing others drinking. Techniques of coping included avoiding certain situations and setting goals that entailed distracting attention away from the desire to drink. Angela recognized that the mornings were when she most craved alcohol. A walking activity was agreed requiring Angela to engage in a warm-up exercise routine before leaving the house and then taking a walk every morning. The exact route was discussed and agreed and the time, distance and duration of the walk determined. This time and distance was increased weekly over a three-week period with each session being noted in the diary alongside notes recording mood state, and feelings of anxiety/confidence before and after each session. At the end of each week Angela outlined in her diary perceived gains from her exercise participation and any perceived losses. Examples of gains included feeling fitter – less out of breath, feeling warm and relaxed, enhanced feeling of well-being, doing something good with my body. Losses included feeling tired and getting bored with the activity. She listed more gains than losses, indicating her commitment to the exercise regimen; whenever she felt an urge to return to drinking she was encouraged to use these gains to think about the positive benefits. If she had noted more losses than gains then it would have been important to look at the losses and to see if these could be overcome. For example in relation to boredom the possibility of identifying a walking buddy could have been discussed. The easy-to-follow warm-up exercises were illustrated in a handout which also included muscular endurance exercises for strength and stretching exercises; these were undertaken following the aerobic walking session. This activity was undertaken by Angela to increase her confidence about returning to an exercise class and/or participating in an established locally run walking group.

Angela also attended weekly group sessions with other problem drinkers where interpersonal skills in dealing with conflict resolution, rational thinking and problem solving were explored. Angela became aware that she had a very limited social network that left her feeling isolated; she also became aware of her lack of confidence, which prevented her taking up opportunities of vocational training. These sessions, aimed at increasing social skills, involved modelling, role-play and practising newly acquired social skills in real-life situations where excessive drinking is a possible risk.

Treating the cognitive element

Angela's beliefs, patterns of thinking, assumptions and expectations that are related to drinking and her alcohol-related problems were explored in order that she could be explicitly aware of them and the subsequent impact on her behaviour. Cognitive restructuring allowed Angela to recognize the way that her emotions, thoughts and feelings had influenced her drinking behaviour in the past, leading to alcohol-related problems. Firstly, Angela learned to recognize the negative thoughts that she frequently rehearsed as antecedents, beliefs and consequences to excessive drinking. The process of engagement during the interview was similar to that outlined in detail in Chapter 5. Angela recorded in her diary her negative thoughts and her self-talk around situations where she either was craving for a drink or engaged in drinking. Through this process of self-monitoring Angela was able to come to an understanding of the relationship between her thinking and her problematic drinking. Once this was achieved the next step was to learn how to interrupt the stream of negative thoughts and by challenging those thoughts to eventually lead to new ways of interpreting the situation. This process was enhanced by engaging in group sessions with other problem drinkers where previously held beliefs, expectations and causal influences around drinking were challenged by individuals in the group. Challenging negative thinking is based on identifying cognitive errors, for example 'alcohol addiction is a disease and I cannot help my behaviour'. This can be reinterpreted by thinking about other interpretations and explanations, exploring the evidence and looking at distortions in thinking. For Angela, using her diary to review experiences where she was successful in coping was helpful in changing her negative thoughts and beliefs. Using her diary, Angela managed to provide convincing evidence that she was becoming more confident about her physical appearance and feeling good about herself, by gradually exposing herself to high-risk drinking situations she gained confidence that her negative thoughts were changing and that she was able to demonstrate newly gained social skills to deal with the situation.

After participating for nine weeks in the walking programme, Angela felt confident to attend her local gym which was accessed through a GP referral scheme. This led to new social contacts and at six-month review Angela had maintained her abstinence, had made new friends and had enrolled in a computer training course at her local further education college. Angela has gained confidence in reducing the risk of relapse by putting in place a relapse emergency procedure (Parks et al 2001). She carries a reminder card which outlines steps she should take in the event of returning to drinking; this includes the contact number of a friend who has agreed to support her in the eventuality of relapse, and of her key worker from the drug and alcohol rehabilitation unit.

Conclusion

There is global evidence that the number of young people who are experiencing social and health-related problems through alcohol abuse is on the increase. The reason for this increase and the links between alcohol addiction, health and social factors is multifaceted and complex. Cognitive–behavioural approaches to the treatment of alcohol abuse and dependence offer a number of useful strategies that have been found to be effective in controlling drinking and in assisting clients to attain and maintain abstinence. The strategies outlined in this chapter provide an introduction to the topic for health-care professionals and students. Undertaking training and experience in using these strategies is recommended in order to establish a range of skills that will allow the correct selection and integration of techniques to meet the different needs of clients. Occupational therapists and physiotherapists can enhance their professional skills by engaging in this training and by using these approaches alongside their traditional roles in the treatment of people with alcohol addiction.

117

 ## Key Messages

- Problem drinking is on the increase, especially for young people and women.
- Changing patterns of alcohol consumption are leading to increased morbidity and mortality at an earlier age.
- Learning theory and social learning theory have directly influenced CBT approaches to the treatment of addiction.
- Efficacy for CBT in the treatment of alcohol dependence is modest.
- Exercise may be a useful adjunct to CBT in the treatment of alcohol dependence, improving fitness and lifestyle change.
- CBT in combination with opiate antagonists SSRIs is beneficial in reducing relapse rates.

References

American Psychiatric Association 1994
Diagnostic and Statistical Manual of Mental
Disorders, 4th edn. American Psychiatric
Association, Washington, DC

Anderson P, Baumberg B 2006 Alcohol in
Europe. http://ec.europe.eu/health-eu/news
alcoholineurope en.htm

Angelone S M, Bellini L, di Bella D et al 1998
Effects of fluvoxamine and citalopram in
maintaining abstinence in a sample of Italian
detoxified alcoholics. Alcohol and Alcoholism
33:341–345

Annis H 1986 A relapse prevention model
for the treatment of alcoholics. In: Miller W,
Rollnick S (eds) Motivational interviewing:
preparing people to change addictive behaviour. Plenum, New York, pp 407–431

Anton R F, Moak D H, Waid R et al 1999 Naltrexone and cognitive behavioural therapy for
the treatment of outpatient alcoholics: results of
a placebo-controlled trial. American Journal of
Psychiatry 156(11):1758–1764

Bandura A 1986 Social foundations of thought
and action: a social cognitive theory. Prentice
Hall, Englewood Cliffs, NJ

Bandura A 1997 Self efficacy: the exercise of
control. W H Freeman, San Francisco, CA

Baucom D H, Shoham V, Mueser K T et al 1998
Empirically supported couple and family
interventions for marital distress and adult
mental health problems. Journal of Consulting
and Clinical Psychology 66(1):53–88

Bukstein O G, Trunzo A C 2005 Alcohol use
disorder in adolescents. Minerva Paediatrica
57(1):7–20

Coleman L, Cater S 2005 Underage 'risky'
drinking. Joseph Rowntree Foundation, New
York

Conason A H, Sher L 2006 Alcohol use in
adolescents with eating disorders. International
Journal of Adolescent Medicine and Health
18(1):31–36

Cutler R B, Fishbain D A 2005 Are alcoholism
treatments effective? Project MATCH data BMC
Public Health (Electronic Resource) 5:75

Donaghy M E 1997 The investigation of
exercise as an adjunct to the treatment and
rehabilitation of the problem drinker. PhD
Thesis, Faculty of Medicine, Glasgow University

Donaghy M E, Mutrie N 1999 Is exercise
beneficial in the treatment and rehabilitation of
the problem drinker? A critical review. Physical
Therapy Reviews 4:153–166

Donaghy M E, Ussher M 2005 Exercise
interventions in drug and alcohol
rehabilitation. In: Faulkener G, Taylor A H
(eds) Exercise in health and mental health:
emerging relationships. Routledge, London
pp 46–89

Donovan D M, Marlatt G A 1988 Assessment of
addictive behaviours. Guilford, New York

Feeney G F, Connor J P, Young R M et al 2004
Alcohol dependence: the impact of cognitive
behavioural therapy with or without
naltrexone on subjective health status. The
Australian and New Zealand Journal of
Psychiatry 38(10):842–848

Franken I H A, Rosso M, Van Honk J 2003
Selective memory for alcohol cues in alcoholics
and its relation to craving. Cognitive Therapy
and Research 27(4):481–488

Havassy B, Hall S, Wasserman D 1991 Social
support and relapse: commonalities among
alcoholics, opiate users, and cigarette smokers.
Addictive Behaviours 16:235–246

Heather N, Tebbutt J 1989 The effectiveness
of treatment for alcohol and drug problems:
an overview. Monograph series No 11,
National Campaign against Drug Abuse,
Government Publishing Service, Canberra,
Australia

Hibell B, Andersson B, Bjarnason T et al 2004
The ESPAD Report 2003: alcohol and other
drug use among students in 35 European
countries. Stockholm, Sweden, The Swedish
Council for Information on Alcohol and Other
Drugs (CAN) and the Pompidou Group at the
Council of Europe. www.espad.org

Honess T, Seymour L, Webster R 2000 The
social contexts of underage drinking. London:
The Research Development and Statistics
Directorate, the Home Office. http://www.
homeoffice.gov.uk/rds/pdfs/occ-drink.pdf

Irvin J E, Bowers C A, Dunn M E et al 1999
Efficacy of relapse prevention: a meta-analytic
review. Journal of Consulting and Clinical
Psychology 67(4):563–570

Kassel J D, Wagner E F, Unrod M 1999
Alcoholism behaviour therapy. In: Hersen M,
Bellack A S (eds) Handbook of comparative
interventions for adult disorders, 2nd edn. John
Wiley, pp 626–651

Klingemann H, Gmel G 2001 Alcohol and its social consequences – the forgotten dimension. Kluwer Academic Publishers on behalf of WHO-EURO, Dordrecht, Netherlands

Long C G, Williams M, Midgley M et al 2000 Within-program factors as predictors of drinking outcome following cognitive-behavioural treatment Addictive Behaviours 25(4):573–578

Longabaugh R, Donovan D M, Karno M P et al 2005 Active ingredients: how and why evidence-based alcohol behavioural treatment interventions work. Alcoholism: Clinical and Experimental Research 29(2):235–247

Lowman C, Allen J, Stout R L 1996 Replication and extension of Marlatt's taxonomy of relapse precipitants: overview of procedures and results. The Relapse Research Group Addiction 91(suppl):51–71

Marlatt G A 1996 Taxonomy of high-risk situations for alcohol relapse: evolution and development of cognitive-behavioural model. Addiction 91(suppl):37–49

Marlatt G A, Gordon J R 1985 Relapse prevention: maintenance strategies in the treatment of addictive behaviours. Guilford, New York

Meyers R J, Smith J E 1997 Getting off the fence: procedures to engage treatment resistant drinkers. Journal of Substance Abuse Treatment 14(5):467–472

Miller W R 1983 Motivational interviewing with problem drinkers. Behavioural Psychotherapy 11:147–172

Miller W R, Hester R K 1995 Treatment for alcohol problems: toward an informed eclecticism. In: Handbook of alcoholism treatment approaches: effective alternatives, 2nd edn. Allyn & Bacon, Needham Heights, MA, pp 1–11

Miller W R, Longabaugh R 2003 Summary and conclusions in treatment matching in alcoholism. In: Babor T F, Del Boca F K (eds) Cambridge University Press, pp 207–221

Miller W R, Rollnick S 1991 Motivational interviewing: preparing people to change addictive behaviours. Guilford, New York

Miller W R, Westerberg V S, Harris R J et al 1996 What predicts relapse? Prospective testing and antecedent models. Addiction 91(suppl): S155–S171

Morgenstern J, Longabaugh R 2000 Cognitive-behavioral treatment for alcohol dependence: a review of evidence for its hypothesized mechanisms of action. Addiction 95(10):1475–1490

Nationmaster 2004 Nationmaster countries by mortality. www.nationmaster.com/ graph-T/mor alc liv dis (accessed 5 Sept 2006)

Office of National Statistics 2005a General household survey. www.statistics.gov.uk

Office of National Statistics 2005b Mortality and morbidity. www.statistics.gov.uk

O'Leary T A, Monti P M 2002 Cognitive-behavioral therapy for alcohol addiction. In: Hoffman S G, Tompson M C (eds) Treating chronic and severe mental disorders: a handbook of empirically supported interventions. Guilford Press, pp 234–257

Orford J 1985 Excessive appetites: a psychological view of addiction. Wiley & Sons, Chichester

Parks G A, Anderson B K, Marlatt G A 2001 Relapse prevention therapy. In: Heather N, Peters T J, Stockwell T (eds) Alcohol dependence and problems. Wiley & Sons, Chichester, pp 575–592

Polich J, Armour D. Braiker H 1980 The course of alcoholism: four years after treatment. Rand Corporation, Santa Monica, CA

Prochaska J, Diclemente C 1986 Towards a comprehensive model of change. In: Miller W, Heather N (eds) Treating addictive behaviours. Plenum Press, New York, pp 3–27

Prochaska J O, Diclemente C C 1992 Stages of change in the modification of problem behaviours. In: Hersen M, Eisler R, Miller P (eds) Progress in behaviour modification 28:183–218, Sycamore Publishing, Sycamore, IL

Project MATCH 1997 Matching alcoholism treatments to client heterogeneity: Project MATCH post treatment drinking outcomes. Journal of Studies on Alcohol 58:7–29

Project MATCH 1998 Matching alcoholism treatments to client heterogeneity: Project MATCH three-year drinking outcomes. Alcoholism, Clinical and Experimental Research 22(6):300–1311

Rehm, J, Room R, Monteiro M et al 2004 Alcohol. In: Ezzati M, Lopez A D, Rogers A et al (eds) Comparative quantification of health risks: global and regional burden of disease due to selected major risk factors. WHO, Geneva

Rollnick S, Allison J 2001 Motivational interviewing. In: Heather N, Peters T J, Stockwell T (eds) Alcohol dependence and problems. Wiley and Sons, Chichester, pp 593–603

Royal College of Physicians 2001 Alcohol: can the NHS afford it? Recommendations for a coherent alcohol strategy for hospitals. Royal College of Physicians: Sarum Colour View Group, Salisbury

Saunders B 1994 The cognitive-behavioural approach to the management of addictive behaviour. In: Chick J, Cantwell, R (eds) Alcohol and drug misuse. College Seminar Series, Royal College of Psychiatrists, London, pp 156–173

Saunders B, Allsop S 1991 Incentives and restraints: clinical research into problem drug use and self control. In: Heather N, Miller W, Greeley J (eds) Self control and the addictive behaviours. Pergamon Press, Sydney, pp 283–303

Sobell M B, Sobell L C 1993 Problem drinkers: guided self-change treatment. Guilford, New York

Trimpey J 1989 Rational recovery from alcoholism: the small book, 3rd edn. Lotus Press, Lotus, CA

Wiers R W, Cox W M, Fadardi J S et al 2006 The search for new ways to change implicit alcohol-related cognitions in heavy drinkers. Alcoholism, Clinical and Experimental Research 30(2):320–331

World Health Organization 2004 Global status report on alcohol. WHO, Geneva

World Health Organization 2005 Alcohol policy in the WHO European region: current status and the way forward. WHO Regional Office for Europe, Copenhagen

Chronic pain
Denis Martin and Liz Macleod

8

Introduction

Chronic pain is one of the most significant long-term conditions in terms of its negative personal, social and economic impact. A major survey in the Grampian area of Scotland estimated that as many as one person in every seven directly experiences significant problems because of chronic pain (Elliott et al 1999). As well as pain there is compromised function and social participation and for many people this causes them severe problems, including problems in areas such as employment and relationships. For those who value the importance of an issue in economic terms, it is estimated that days lost at work due to back pain alone account for £12 billion per year, equivalent to 22% of the UK health-care expenditure and 1.5% of the gross domestic product (Dr Foster 2004). Despite the degree and nature of the problem it is not being adequately addressed by the NHS at primary- or secondary-care levels (Dr Foster 2004, CSAG 2000). Chronic pain is an example of a lived-in long-term condition (Christianson et al 1998). A lived-in long-term condition is one to which people need to adapt to live with for the rest of their lives and for which there is, as yet, no cure. It is now accepted that health care for people with chronic pain and, indeed, other long-term conditions that they will live with for the rest of their lives, is in need of a system change (Christianson et al 1998, Von Korff et al 2002). The problem is that up until now health care has been driven by biomedical models that work well with conditions for which there *is* an obtainable cure. For the management of long-term conditions in which there is, as yet, *no cure*, these models are outdated and fundamentally inconsistent with the needs of people at personal and population levels.

The biopsychosocial model

From a biomedical stance, pain is viewed as a sensory phenomenon associated with actual tissue damage and it is thus treated as a symptom of an underlying injury or disease. While this may be a useful working paradigm for acute pain, it is too narrow to capture the complexities involved in chronic pain. Consequently, strategies for managing chronic pain have been adopted and developed around a biopsychosocial approach (Keefe et al 2004). The biopsychosocial model provides a wider perspective on pain in the context of a dynamic interplay among physiological, psychological and environmental factors (Hanson & Gerber 1989). It does not restrict pain to requiring association with actual tissue damage, and it encompasses the emotional aspects of pain as well as the sensory. Therefore, it is in line with current definitions of pain as *an unpleasant sensory and emotional experience associated with actual or potential tissue damage, or described in terms of such damage* (Merskey & Bogduk 1994).

The biopsychosocial approach recognizes that the impact of pain has influence at physiological, psychological and environmental levels and, in turn, that the impact of pain is influenced from each of these levels. The biopsychosocial approach fits well with contemporary ideas about disability and function as described by the WHO International Classification of Function, Disability and Health (ICF) (WHO 2001). The ICF is built on ideas of body structures and functions, and activity and participation (Figure 8.1). Body structures include the nervous system and anatomical parts involved in movement. Body functions include sensation, cognitive processes and motor skills. Activity refers to the capacity of an individual to carry out a task and participation describes what an individual actually does as a social being. In the language of the ICF, problems with body structures and body functions are described as impairments, problems with capacity are activity limitations, and problems with performance are described as restrictions on participation. The ICF also discusses the importance of personal factors (e.g. age, sex, coping styles and experience) and environmental factors (e.g. social support and attitudes, policies and technology).

The ICF replaces the previous WHO model (the ICIDH – the International Classification of Impairments, Disabilities and Handicaps), which was generally interpreted as describing a linear progression from injury/disease to restricted ability and activity and, ultimately, to reduced social participation. It also gives more explicit and substantial recognition to the importance of environment and context. Already,

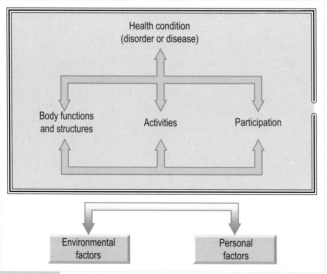

Figure 8.1 ● WHO (2001) International Classification of Functioning, Disability and Health.

the applicability of the ICF has been demonstrated in chronic pain (Steiner et al 2002), low-back pain (Soukup & Vollestad 2001, Chwastiak & Von Korff 2003) and rheumatoid arthritis (Fransen et al 2002).

Thoughts and feelings

People with chronic pain experience many feelings. Those that are commonly reported are anger, frustration, anxiety, low mood and depression. Many people with chronic pain also commonly report that they have recurring thoughts such as:

- Why me?
- Is there no end to this pain?
- I can't handle this pain any more.
- Why have I allowed myself to get into this state?

Often this thinking becomes so ingrained that people don't realize that it is happening. These are all negative thoughts and feelings, and while they are often problematic for people with chronic pain it is worth pointing out that they are perfectly normal and are not surprising given that someone has chronic pain.

The problem is that these negative thoughts can lead to more negative feelings, and the negative feelings can lead to more negative thoughts. The negative thoughts and feelings can reinforce negative behaviour such as inactivity, aggression and withdrawing from social contact – destructive behaviours, which make things worse for the person with chronic pain.

Cognitive–behavioural therapy

Recognition of the relationships among thoughts, feelings and behaviour explains why progressive thinking holds that the management of chronic pain should be underpinned by cognitive–behavioural principles (Harding & Williams 1995, Morley 2004). This thinking comes from evidence and a history of developing practice that cognitive–behavioural therapy is an effective method of helping some people to live with their pain as active participants in society. Cognitive–behavioural therapy operates from a fundamental basis that it has a role to play in helping people to break the damaging cycle of interactions among negative thoughts, feelings and behaviour that is a feature of many people who are experiencing difficulties with chronic pain (and other long-term conditions). The approach was informed by people like Beck (1967) and Bandura (1977, 1997) who presented ideas about the links between maladaptive negative thinking and unhelpful behaviour in health. Beck, focusing on depression, proposed that therapy should target negative thinking through increasing people's understanding of their condition and by guiding them to re-evaluate their negative thoughts about behaviour in the light of having actually carried out that behaviour. Bandura described the idea of self-efficacy in which behaviour is influenced by a person's confidence in their ability to do something. These and similar ideas have been shown to be relevant in the management of chronic pain.

For example, negative thoughts and feelings that are commonly associated with chronic pain are seen to reinforce behaviours that are not helpful.

Catastrophizing is an extreme manifestation of negative thinking that is common in people who are having difficulty in managing chronic pain (Sullivan et al 1997). Basically, catastrophizing is an exaggeration of the likelihood of the worst possible scenario happening, combined with a lack of faith about the likelihood of being able to do anything about it.

Fear avoidance, or kinesiophobia, is another common manifestation of negative thinking that has a detrimental influence on behaviour (Vlaeyen & Linton 2000). Here, people associate a high risk of damage with movement and, therefore, avoid performing activities, leading to further problems, including deconditioning. As discussed in Chapter 1, a response like avoidance of feared movement may be reinforced by anxiety. Even when misplaced beliefs about damage associated with feared movement are addressed the avoidance behaviour may need to be unlearnt through graded exposure to movement accompanied with relaxation. Fear avoidance is mostly a feature of chronic pain, often back pain, associated with an injurious incident: in chronic pain associated with overuse it is argued that the concept is less relevant (Vlaeyen & Morley 2004).

Specific aims of cognitive–behavioural therapy include helping people with chronic pain to:

- Recognize negative thoughts and feelings
- Understand the problems with negative thoughts and feelings
- Challenge negative thoughts and behaviours
- Develop positive ways of acting through techniques such as relaxation, pacing and goal setting.

Problem solving is important. The person with chronic pain assumes the role of an expert in their own condition and works together with the therapist to identify specific problems and come up with practical solutions. Cognitive–behavioural therapy encourages people to be active participants in their health care, becoming knowledgeable about chronic pain and its impact and ultimately taking control of the pain rather than letting pain control them.

A simplified example of a negative cycle is:

Everyone is going to the seaside. You tell yourself: 'I can't drive to the seaside as it is two hours away and I can't sit that long.' You have the experience of having driven to the seaside and spending three days in bed afterwards with a flare-up. You don't drive to the seaside. You feel miserable about not being able to drive to the seaside, you feel left out, hopeless and depressed.

A simplified example of challenging this negative cycle is:

You tell yourself: 'I can't drive to the seaside as it is two hours away and I can't sit that long.' Then you tell yourself: 'I can't sit for two hours but if I stop every 40 minutes or so I can drive to the seaside.' You feel good about going to the seaside. You drive to the seaside with a few stops on the way. You feel good at having driven to the seaside and having been part of the family outing.

Recognizing and challenging negative self-talk is not easy. It is a skill and it needs practice. Like all skills, while some people can pick it up by themselves, many others need help. Health professionals can help by offering guidance to the person with chronic pain, challenging their misconceptions and negative thinking patterns. As discussed in Chapter 1, the above techniques are thought to be best used within a cognitive framework.

Education

Education is a fundamental part of pain management. It is important that people with chronic pain are able to access appropriate information and understand it in relation to their own particular circumstances to address misplaced beliefs about pain. Education can be effective in reducing pain-related disability and as a support into self-management for people with chronic pain (Moseley 2004, Burton et al 1999).

Because thoughts and feelings are susceptible to external environmental influences, education of family, friends, work colleagues and carers is also important (Ferrell & Ferrell 1991).

Pacing and goal setting

People who have benefited from pain management often state that pacing and goal setting are among the most useful skills that they have acquired (Martin et al 2004). Pacing and goal setting are useful techniques to help people to exercise and improve activity and participation (Harding & Williams 1995, Fey & Fordyce 1983).

Many different forms of exercise are put forward as being helpful for people with chronic pain. A recent systematic review of the literature points to a conclusion that exercise, in whatever form, is worth trying and that it may have long-lasting benefits (Liddle et al 2004). The review, which focused on physiotherapy, also stated that supervision can improve the outcomes of exercise for people with chronic pain (Liddle et al 2004). An unfortunate feature of chronic pain is that some people overdo exercise and activity when they feel active. They continue with activities until reaching the limits of their physical capacity, which often results in fatigue and flare-up of pain that, in turn, leads to prolonged down-time. Flare-up has been compared to breakthrough pain seen in cases of cancer (Svendsen et al 2005). When the flare-up is over, the person feels somewhat better and there is a tendency to try to compensate for lost time by overdoing things once more. The probability of subsequent flare-up is high. The typical overactivity/underactivity cycle is harmful because its natural progression is towards prolonged inactivity. Pacing is used to smooth out the excessive peaks and troughs of overactivity and underactivity and help the patient find a level of activity that they can be confident of managing without flare-up of pain. The underlying concept of pacing is to replace activity that is guided by capacity and motivation with activity guided by predetermined quota. The skills of pacing are, therefore, to determine tolerances – the amount of activity that becomes problematic; to set baselines for actions well within the tolerance limits; and to intersperse baseline activity with rest from that action. It is useful at the start of therapy to help the person find the baselines for sitting, standing and walking so that these can be integrated into everyday activity. There are, of course, many other different actions with varying importance for different people. The aim of operating with baselines in mind is to make tasks more achievable.

Tolerances and baselines are defined in quantifiable dimensions – usually time or distance. For example, in terms of time, sitting tolerance would be how long someone can sit before becoming fatigued and/or before the pain flares up. A complicating factor is that often these consequences of carrying out the action for too long are not felt immediately – there may be a delay until the next day. Thus, in the process of determining tolerances and baselines, there is often a period of exploration and trial and error, and it is beneficial for the person to receive guidance. This is an important role for the therapist when discussing exercise and activity. Having decided on the tolerance level, the next step is to calculate an appropriate baseline – in this case a time for sitting that is well within the limits of the tolerance time. Opinions vary and the calculation can be arbitrary but some practitioners recommend setting baselines at 50% of tolerance, while others may recommend 80%. In summary, pacing is about finding a balance between doing too much and doing too little, being too active and not being active enough. The skill helps people to learn to get into a pattern of operating in small chunks of activity interspersed with regular breaks from that activity (Nielson et al 2001).

Alongside pacing, goal setting can be useful in helping people with chronic pain to carry out tasks and take part in activities like work and social events that otherwise they can find difficult. Goal setting involves defining aims and setting targets to achieve. Goal setting is a skill and, again, many people require guidance. Very often, for example, people with chronic pain set goals that are too difficult to achieve in time. This causes problems because when people can't achieve their goal they can become frustrated and give up trying. Another problem is that often people with chronic pain set goals that are unclear. It is then impossible to say if they have been achieved or not. Thus a role of therapists is to guide the person to develop goals that are SMART – Specific, Measurable, Activity-related, Realistic, Time-related:

- Specific means that the goal is very clearly defined. Wanting to dance is not specific. Wanting to dance for ten minutes with the groom's father at your daughter's wedding is a more specific goal.
- Measurable means that it is clear when the goal has been achieved.
- Activity-related means that the goal involves actually doing something.
- Realistic means that the goal is possible. There are many things other than chronic pain that can stop the achievement of a goal, such as lack of finance.
- Time-related means that a date is set by which time the goal should be achieved.

The therapist works with the person to help to divide the goal into smaller mini-goals. The person is rewarded with success in reaching the mini-goal while at the same time advancing towards the overall goal. Goal setting is helped by feedback from the therapist.

Within pacing and goal setting, the therapist can offer guidance on improving activity and participation by the use of such skills as prioritizing of tasks, delegating and planning ahead. Opinion based on research to date is that cognitive–behavioural therapy is of value for people with chronic pain (Vlaeyen & Morley 2005, Keefe et al 2004, Morley 2004). For example, a systematic review of randomized controlled trials concluded that cognitive–behavioural therapy was beneficial in the dimensions of pain experience, thoughts and feelings, behaviour and social function (Morley et al 1999). Other systematic reviews (van Tulder et al 2000, Guzman et al 2001) indicate that cognitive–behavioural approaches are of use in chronic pain management.

Vlaeyen and Morley (2005) point to four areas that require more investigation:

- People who do not respond to therapy
- Improving the magnitude of the effect of therapy (described as similar to that of CBT for other conditions – quite modest)
- Attributing specific outcomes to specific aspects of therapy
- Finding out more about the basic biological–behavioural mechanisms involved in chronic pain.

There are a number of difficulties in providing research evidence to support the use of CBT for management of chronic pain. CBT contains different elements, and the amount and contribution of these depend on the different systems of delivery (Morley 2004, van Tulder et al 2000). Thus it is extremely difficult to state conclusively which part or parts of the therapy are responsible for which outcome or outcomes. Also it is difficult to standardize the component parts of the therapy. These and other problems, however, do not have to stand in the way of investigation. Alongside the usual range of research methods, other methods of investigation such as cross-lagged panel designs (Burns et al 2003) and clinical practice improvement methodology (Horn 2001) have potential to address these questions.

127

Pain management programmes

The use of cognitive–behavioural therapy for people with chronic pain can be seen alongside the rise in popularity of pain management programmes. These were first developed in the 1960s in the USA by some pioneering doctors who realized that their usual methods of treating pain were not meeting the needs of many of their patients. Pain management programmes spread internationally and have been provided in the UK since the 1980s. A distinctive feature of pain management programmes is that the focus is on *the impact of pain* rather than just pain itself. This is an important distinction that goes beyond mere semantics. While any reduction in pain is welcomed, the main aims of pain management revolve around helping people to develop ways to overcome disabling effects of chronic pain. While other approaches have the primary aim of reducing or removing pain, pain management programmes set out to help people to learn skills to deal with the distress and disabling effects of chronic pain. The programmes are multidisciplinary. The British Pain Society recommends pain management programmes (British Pain Society 2003). Ideally they should be staffed by a doctor specializing in pain management, a clinical psychologist, a physiotherapist, an occupational therapist and a nurse. Some pain management programmes link up with vocational trainers to try to help people regain or retain employment (Watson et al 2004). Education is a major feature of pain management programmes and it tends to address:

* Mechanisms of pain and its effects
* The differences between acute and chronic pain
* Stress and pain
* Dealing with the psychological effects of chronic pain
* Exercise
* Pacing and goal setting
* Drugs and medicines
* Sleep.

As well as education, people receive training and practice on the following strategies and skills:

* Coming to terms with the reality of chronic pain
* Improvement of fitness, mobility and posture
* Overcoming fear of movement
* Development of ways to cope with stress, anxiety, depression and anger
* Relaxation techniques
* Getting back to everyday activities
* Making best use of medication
* Making best use of aids and equipment
* Improving communication with health professionals
* Improving communication with friends and family.

The content and delivery of pain management programmes can vary but they do have shared characteristics. The programmes are usually run, on an outpatient or inpatient basis, for groups of 8–14 people with chronic pain. The British Pain Society recommends that outpatient pain management programmes should last between 6–8 weeks. Within this period people should attend for 1–2 sessions per week. Each session should last for 2–3 hours. Further recommendations are that inpatient pain management programmes should comprise around 15 days and that these 15 days should happen within a 3–4 week period (to allow for days off).

In the UK, pain management programmes are not available in every part of the country. Waiting lists are long and systematic long-term support is not a common feature. Increasingly, pain management is being delivered beyond this format, for example, in primary care (Von Korff 2005) and in the voluntary sector (Martin et al 2004). These initiatives have the potential to provide cost-effective access to a larger number of people. Strong arguments have been put forward in support of systematic integration of the various sectors (Christianson et al 1998, Von Korff et al 2002). The potential advantage of this is that people would be less likely to receive mixed messages and conflicting information about chronic pain, and it would provide a more adequate framework for long-term support and use of health and social care. Through custom and practice cognitive–behavioural therapy for chronic pain has been seen to be the territory of clinical psychologists. Increasingly, it is becoming accepted that cognitive–behavioural principles can be applied by others, and a growing number of nurses, physiotherapists, occupational therapists and other health professionals are using the principles of cognitive–behavioural therapy in their management of people with chronic pain (Harding & Williams 1995, LeFort et al 1998, Johnstone et al 2003). See Case Study 8.1. This is not yet standard practice throughout each of the professions, however, and the need for improvements in education have been highlighted (Jones et al 2000).

CASE STUDY 8.1

Jane is a 35-year-old woman who works as an office assistant. Her case has been selected to illustrate benefit from a cognitive–behavioural approach to pain management that was delivered mainly by a physiotherapist with input from occupational therapy and clinical psychology.

Her initial assessment revealed that she had had back pain over two years. She attributed her problems to a painful episode of lifting a box at work. She continued to work after the episode and during this time she had frequent periods of time off because of difficulty in managing her pain. She also had numerous investigations. At this stage she had been off work for four months although she was still an employee.

X-rays showed some arthritic changes at L3/4/5 and there were signs of a small bulging disc between L4 and L5. She had constant, variable pain in her lower back with occasional leg pain. Her neck and shoulders were painful now too. She was also slightly asthmatic.

She was living alone in her own flat. Jane's elderly parents lived nearby. She was their only child, and they were very concerned about her and were actively doing lots to try to help her. For example, her father always drove her to appointments as Jane would only drive as far as her parents' home, which was two streets away. Also, her mother had taken it upon herself to do all of the housework for her.

Jane said that while she had a couple of good friends she was not particularly outgoing. She was noticeably overweight and said that she had always been so, although she had put on extra weight in the last few years. She described herself as living a quiet life that was mostly sedentary. Her main activities were walking and shopping, plus she would occasionally go swimming. Since experiencing pain, she had reduced these activities considerably.

The physiotherapist observed that she was very anxious. She described herself as 'panicky' and said that she had always been anxious. She also said that she was hard working and conscientious and her standard of work had always been appreciated by her colleagues. Her manager had reassured her verbally that her job would remain open for her return but Jane did not think that he had much understanding of what she was experiencing. Her manager was contacting her frequently with enquiries about when she planned to return to work. Jane said that she would like to return but she saw no way forward until the pain settled down. She pointed out that most of her time at work was spent in sitting and that worried her because sitting was painful. She was also very anxious about having to do things that involved bending and carrying objects like files.

Jane stated that her problems were due to 'a slipped disc' and arthritis in her back and thus she had decided to avoiding lifting, housework and shopping or anything that she thought would cause further damage to her back.

In the assessment she also completed some outcome measures: Tampa Scale of Kinesiophobia (TSK) (Vlaeyen et al 1995); Sickness Impact Profile (SIP) (Bergner et al 1981) Pain Self Efficacy Questionnaire (PSEQ) (Nicholas et al 1992); Five minute walk test (Harding et al 1994). These showed:

PSEQ 25/60 (a low score indicates low self-efficacy)
SIP 15/24 (a high score indicates reduced function)
TSK 45/51 (a high score indicates problems with fear avoidance)
Five minute walking distance = 112 metres

Jane's main problems centred around:

- Fear avoidance
- Lack of assertiveness with her parents and manager
- Deconditioning
- General anxiety

The plan of management was as follows. The differences between chronic pain and acute pain were explained. Jane was guided through information that included fairly complex issues such as sensitization and the influence of stress on chronic pain. The physiotherapist discussed this information with Jane as well as her beliefs about arthritis and damage to intervertebral discs 'producing' her chronic pain. A consistent feature of the discussion was the physiotherapist challenging Jane's beliefs about her pain and thinking patterns. The physiotherapist discussed with her the principles of managing, controlling and negotiating with pain, introducing Jane to the contrast between hurt and harm. The physiotherapist was aware that Jane, since her original injury, had held the belief that her pain had to be associated with tissue damage. Although this thinking shifted over the course of their discussions, any indication that Jane was defaulting to her original belief was gently challenged and reinforcement of her efforts to make change was applauded. They discussed the importance of exercise in increasing her fitness with a view to becoming more active. Jane was helped to come to terms with the idea that her condition is a long-term one with a view to promoting her confidence in her ability to manage it.

Having been helped to understand the importance of activity and overcoming deconditioning, Jane agreed to increase her activity levels. Pacing and goal setting were explained and, with guidance from the physiotherapist, she agreed to identify tolerances and set baselines, initially for sitting and walking. As she progressed, she developed specific goals related to driving, housework and swimming and, again with guidance from the physiotherapist, she identified tolerances and developed baselines to help pace these activities. They both agreed on principles that included carrying out activities without pushing through pain and doing activities every day (as well as a daily walk). Jane also agreed that the activities should be done in accordance with a formal plan. The physiotherapist monitored her progress, gave regular feedback and worked with her to review and develop the plan as she progressed. Jane was encouraged to get out and about with her friends. To this end, she decided that it was a good idea to take a friend with her when she went swimming. The physiotherapist's understanding of Jane's chronic anxiety was important in the goal-setting approach. By working collaboratively, they were able to include strategies that helped her achieve her activity goals and manage her anxiety too.

Various relaxation techniques were discussed with the physiotherapist. Jane found the breathing exercises to be particularly useful, and she also used a relaxation tape and learned some basic imagery skills. Great emphasis was placed on incorporating these into all of her activities. Her attention was drawn to the relevance of relaxation to the mechanisms of chronic pain, how it could be used to make movement easier and how it could help her to manage her anxiety. She understood that for her, relaxation was a skill and that it was important that she engaged in regular practice.

She was also encouraged to review her pain behaviour and identify patterns. (She accepted the suggestion that she keep a notebook/diary to help with this.) She was helped to analyse these patterns and look at ways of changing them. This helped her negotiate with her pain in such a way that she felt more in control. She learned how to plan and prioritize to get the best outcome. She became more aware of the potential for flare-up and was taught how to manage better when her pain was worse. With the guidance of her physiotherapist, Jane drew up a written plan of action to help to minimize the negative effect of flare-up. (This preparation is important because it is very difficult to come up with a rational plan of action when the person is experiencing flare-up.)

Through discussions with Jane, it was clear to the therapist that there was a fear-avoidance problem with bending, which was a barrier towards returning to work. They worked through graded exposure to bending and moving (Boersma et al 2004). This was combined with specific work-related goals with a particular focus on carrying files. In addition, the physiotherapist asked her colleague in occupational therapy to help in this area. The occupational therapist helped Jane to recreate, at home, aspects of her office and to practice some of the activities in that modelled environment. This was aimed at strengthening her belief in her ability to work through experience of successfully managing relevant activities. Jane also discussed with the occupational therapist ergonomics and communicating with her manager and work colleagues.

The physiotherapist, while happy to work with Jane in the areas of relaxation and basic imagery, decided to refer her to a clinical psychologist to work on improving her assertiveness. Specifically, both the physiotherapist and the occupational therapist felt that Jane needed to be more assertive with her parents and her work colleagues. Jane was keen to demonstrate that she was a capable worker. She did not like to ask for help and she readily accepted continued requests from her colleagues to take on more work. Her parents' supporting activities tended to be oversolicitous and things like their established practice of insisting on driving her to wherever she needed to go were actually counterproductive to her self-management. The issue was helped by her parents attending a family/carers session. (Jane was fortunate in this case because involvement of the family can be difficult to achieve. An added bonus for Jane was that her manager was persuaded by the occupational therapist to attend the family/carers session to gain more understanding about chronic pain in general and how it affected Jane specifically.)

Finally, at the end of her programme her outcome measures had improved:

PSEQ   50/60
SIP   10/24
TSK   19/51
Five minute walking distance = 198 metres

Jane followed up advice from her physiotherapist and went along to a meeting of the local branch of Pain Association Scotland – a voluntary organization providing support and training in skills of pain management for people in the community. She had said that she 'didn't think she was a group kind of person' but her initial reticence was soon overcome and she was interested to hear the experiences of others. (This is consistent with reports of others who have benefited from this kind of service, e.g. Subramaniam et al 1999). The group also provided a supportive environment to maintain the new skills that she had learned and she also picked up some useful practical advice from some of the other group members.

The main outcomes were as follows. She went back to work part time with the agreement of her manager and this progressed to full time over four months. She became more confident about driving herself and she now does her own housework at her own pace. She has an agreement with her parents that they will help her when she requests it. She still has a tendency to fall back into her old anxious state, especially when she is experiencing flare-up, and she also has periods when her worries return about injuring her back because of disc problems. She is, however, alert to this type of thinking and is able to re-evaluate and rationalize her thoughts. Jane considers that pacing and goal setting are two of the most useful skills that she has developed. While she has found that one pain management programme has been sufficient to help her achieve this level of functioning she is aware that a few others that she met at the time have not benefited to the same degree and that they were only really starting to get to grips with the ideas at the end of the programme. She finds that she is helped by attending meetings of her local Pain Association Scotland group, now and again, to catch up with other people with chronic pain and also to 'top up' her pain management skills.

 ## Key Messages

- Chronic pain has a major negative impact at the personal social and economic level.
- Chronic pain fits with a biopsychosocial perspective of function and disability.
- Cognitive–behavioural therapy is considered to be effective for some people with chronic pain.
- Cognitive–behavioural principles can be applied by a range of health professionals in the management of chronic pain.
- The application of cognitive–behavioural principles for the management of chronic pain needs to be incorporated into education and training for health professionals.

References

Bandura A 1977 Self-efficacy: toward a unifying theory of behavioural change. Psychological Review 84:191–215

Bandura A 1997 Self-efficacy: the exercise of control. W H Freeman, New York

Beck A T 1967 Depression: clinical, experimental and theoretical aspects. Harper and Row, New York

Bergner M, Bobbitt R A, Carter W B et al 1981 The Sickness Impact Profile: development and final revision of a health status measure. Medical Care 19:787–805

Boersma K, Linton S, Overmeer T J et al 2004 Lowering fear-avoidance and enhancing function through exposure in vivo: a multiple baseline study across six patients with back pain. Pain 108:8–16

British Pain Society 2003 Draft of desirable criteria for pain management programmes. British Pain Society, London

Burns J W, Kubilus A, Bruehl S et al 2003 Do changes in cognitive factors influence outcome following multidisciplinary treatment for chronic pain? A cross-lagged panel analysis. Journal of Consulting and Clinical Psychology 71:81–91

Burton A, Waddell G, Tillotson K M et al 1999 Information and advice to patients with back pain can have a positive effect. A randomized controlled trial of a novel educational booklet in primary care. Spine 24:2484–2491

Christianson J B, Taylor R, Knutson D 1998 Restructuring chronic illness management: best practices and innovations in team-based treatment. Jossey-Bass, San Francisco

Chwastiak L A, Von Korff M 2003 Disability in depression and back pain: evaluation of the World Health Organization Disability Assessment Schedule (WHO DAS II) in a primary care setting. Journal of Clinical Epidemiology 56:507–514

CSAG 2000 Clinical Standards Advisory Group: services for patients with pain. HMSO, London

Dr Foster 2004 Adult chronic pain management services in primary care research. Dr Foster, London

Elliott A M, Smith B H, Penny K I et al 1999 The epidemiology of chronic pain in the community. Lancet 354:1248–1252

Ferrell B A, Ferrell B R 1991 Pain management at home. Clinics Geriatric Medicine 7: 765–76

Fey S G, Fordyce W E 1983 Behavioral rehabilitation of the chronic pain patient. Annual Review of Rehabilitation 3:32–63

Fransen J, Uebelhart D, Stucki G et al 2002 The ICIDH-2 as a framework for the assessment of functioning and disability in rheumatoid arthritis. Annals of the Rheumatic Diseases 61:225–231

Guzman J, Esmail R, Karjalainen K et al 2001 Multidisciplinary rehabilitation for chronic low back pain: systematic review. British Medical Journal 322:1511–1516

Hanson R W, Gerber K E 1989 Coping with chronic pain: a guide to patient self-management. Guilford, New York

Harding V, Williams A C de C 1995 Extending physiotherapy skills using a psychological approach: cognitive-behavioural management of chronic pain. Physiotherapy 81:681–688

Harding V R, Williams A, Richardson P H et al 1994 The development of a battery of measures for assessing physical functioning of chronic pain patients. Pain 58:367–375

Horn S D 2001 Quality, clinical practice improvement, and the episode of care. Managed Care Quarterly 9:10–24

Johnstone R, Donaghy M, Martin D J 2003 A pilot study of a cognitive-behavioural therapy approach to physiotherapy, for acute low back pain patients, who show signs of developing chronic pain. Advances in Physiotherapy 2:182–188

Jones D, Ravey J, Steedman W 2000 Developing a measure of beliefs and attitudes about chronic non-malignant pain: a pilot study of occupational therapists. Occupational Therapy International 7:232–245

Keefe F J, Rumble M E, Scipio C D et al 2004 Psychological aspects of persistent pain: current state of the science. Journal of Pain 5:195–211

LeFort S M, Gray-Donald K, Rowat K M et al 1998 Randomized controlled trial of a community-based psychoeducation program for the self-management of chronic pain. Pain 74:297–306

Liddle S D, Baxter G D, Gracey J H 2004 Exercise and chronic low back pain: what works? Pain 107:176–190

Martin D J, Jones D, Bates L 2004 Pain management in the community: user and professional perceptions and education. Final report for the National Lotteries Charity Board

Merskey H, Bogduk N 1994 Classification of chronic pain. Seattle: IASP Press

Morley S 2004 Process and change in cognitive behaviour therapy for chronic pain. Pain 109: 205–206

Morley S, Eccleston C, Williams A 1999 Systematic review and meta-analysis of randomized controlled trials of cognitive behaviour therapy and behaviours therapy for chronic pain in adults, excluding headache. Pain 80:1–13

Moseley G L 2004 Evidence for a direct relationship between cognitive and physical change during an education intervention in people with chronic low back pain. European Journal of Pain 8:39–45

133

Nicholas M K, Wilson P H, Goyen J 1992 Comparison of cognitive-behavioral group treatment and an alternative non-psychological treatment for chronic low back pain. Pain 48:339–347

Nielson W R, Jensen M P, Hill M L 2001 An activity pacing scale for the chronic pain coping inventory: development in a sample of patients with fibromyalgia syndrome. Pain 89:111–115

Soukup M G, Vollestad N K 2001 Classification of problems, clinical findings and treatment goals in patients with low back pain using the ICIDH-2 beta-2. Disability and Rehabilitation 23:462–473

Steiner W A, Ryser L, Huber E et al 2002 Use of the ICF model as a clinical problem-solving tool in physical therapy and rehabilitation medicine. Physical Therapy 82:1098–1107

Subramaniam V, Stewart M W, Smith J F 1999 The development and impact of a chronic pain support group: a qualitative and quantitative study. Journal of Pain and Symptom Management 17:376–383

Sullivan MJL, Rouse D, Bishop S et al 1997 Thought suppression, catastrophizing, and pain. Cognitive Therapy and Research 21:555–568

Svendsen K B, Andersen S, Arnason S et al 2005 Breakthrough pain in malignant and non-malignant diseases: a review of prevalence, characteristics and mechanisms. European Journal of Pain 9:195–206

van Tulder M W, Ostelo RWJG, Vlaeyen JWS et al 2000 Behavioural treatment for chronic low back pain. (Cochrane Review). In: The Cochrane Library Issue 2. Oxford: Update Software

Vlaeyen JWS, Linton S J 2000 Fear-avoidance and its consequences in chronic musculoskeletal pain: a state of the art. Pain 85:317–332

Vlaeyen JWS, Morley S 2004 Active despite pain: the putative role of stop-rules and current mood. Pain 110:512–516

Vlaeyen JWS, Morley S 2005 Cognitive-behavioral treatments for chronic pain: what works for whom? Clinical Journal of Pain. Special Topic Series: Cognitive-Behavioral Treatment for Chronic Pain 21:1–8

Vlaeyen J, Kole-Snijders A, Rotteveel A et al 1995 The role of fear of movements/(re)injury in pain disability. Journal of Occupational Rehabilitation 5:363–372

Von Korff M, Glasgow, R E, Sharpe, M 2002 Organising care for chronic illness. British Medical Journal 352:92–94

Von Korff M, Balderson BHK, Saunders K et al 2005 A trial of an activating intervention for chronic back pain in primary care and physical therapy settings. Pain 113:323–330

Watson P J, Booker C K, Moores L et al 2004 Returning the chronically unemployed with low back pain to employment. European Journal of Pain 8:359–369

WHO 2001 International Classification of Functioning, Disability and Health: ICF. WHO, Geneva

Fibromyalgia management using cognitive–behavioural principles

9

A practical approach for therapists
Mick Skelly

Introduction

Fibromyalgia syndrome is a heterogeneous chronic pain condition (Clauw & Crofford 2003) that is thought to be stress related (Crofford & Demitrack 1996, Sherman et al 2000) and highly similar in terms of physiology, psychology, social vulnerability factors and prognosis to chronic fatigue syndrome (Wessely et al 1998) and depression (Raphael et al 2004). It remains a controversial diagnosis (Earnshaw et al 2001) that some regard as primarily a 'culture-bound syndrome' maintained in particular by iatrogenic factors (Hadler 1997, Malleson 2002). (See Table 9.1.)

Since symptoms always include chronic pain with a sensitized nociceptive system, a degree of chronic fatigue and some level of long-term functional impairment, people with fibromyalgia syndrome will inevitably require input from allied health professionals. This should include physiotherapy, occupational therapy and input from a dietitian. Symptoms are likely to include some degree of depression (Hazemeijer & Rasker 2003) impaired mental functioning – often referred to as 'fibrofog' – and some level of emotional lability, all of which can strongly affect cognition and behaviour. For these reasons, many patients with fibromyalgia syndrome, like people with chronic fatigue syndrome, will 'drift' into mental health services. Furthermore, many patients will be thoroughly 'medicalized' and 'fragmented' along Cartesian lines in terms of their beliefs regarding their condition. That is, they are likely to conceptualize fibromyalgia syndrome as a purely 'physical' medical condition to be cured via medical treatment of which they will be passive recipients and may resent any implication that psychosocial factors could play a part. This can be reinforced by physical assessments of muscular abnormalities that might be influenced by ideomotor action (Hyman 1999). The lack of consistency in approaches to treatment and lack of understanding of the psychosocial and physical links may lead some people to feel that the fibromyalgia syndrome is 'all in the mind' and somehow not a 'real' (physical) condition.

Table 9.1 • The diagnostic criteria for fibromyalgia syndrome (FMS)

	Tender points
'The presence of unexplained widespread pain or aching, persistent fatigue, generalized morning stiffness, non-refreshing sleep, and multiple tender points. Most patients with these symptoms have 11 or more tender points. But a variable proportion of otherwise typical patients may have less than 11 tender points at the time of the examination.'	Along the spine in the neck, where the head and neck meet.
	On the upper line of the shoulder, a little less than halfway from the shoulder to the neck.
	Three finger widths, on a diagonal, inward from the last points.
	On the back fairly close to the dimples above the buttocks, a little less than halfway in towards the spine.
FMS 'is part of a wider syndrome encompassing headaches, irritable bladder, dysmenorrhea, cold sensitivity, Raynaud's phenomenon, restless legs, atypical patterns of numbness and tingling, exercise intolerance and complaints of weakness.' The psychological state is often one of (usually reactive) and anxiety.	Below the buttocks, very close to the edge of the thigh, about three finger widths.
	Frontally on the neck, just above the inner edge of the collarbone.
	Still on the neck, a little further out from the last points, about four finger widths down.
	On the inner (palm) side of the lower arm, about three finger widths below the elbow crease.
	On the inner side of the knee, in the 'fat pad'.

From Starlanyl & Copeland 1996, p 9.

The clinical picture may be further confused in that other 'stress-related' conditions may run in 'parallel' to the fibromyalgia syndrome. These can be divergent and include coronary heart disease, and 'auto-immune' conditions such as most rheumatoid conditions. If this were not enough they are likely to be abnormally susceptible to infection for psychoneuroimmunological reasons and more vulnerable to any neurological 'side-effects' from medication due to a stress-related increase in the permeability of the blood–brain barrier. This may also affect the permeability of intestines alongside raised levels of substance-P and other inflammatory substances since these are higher in both chronic pain conditions and in depression (Carli et al 2000, Raphael et al 2004). There is, therefore, a probable increased risk of irritable bowel syndrome, in the fibromyalgia syndrome, chronic fatigue syndrome and depression patient groups.

There is no clear medical treatment. Despite this, antidepressants may be used and if the pain is severe the patient may be on opiates. With all the other conditions, plus a probable search of several 'health food' shops, patients may be on a cocktail of medications, herbal remedies and the like. Fibromyalgia syndrome sufferers have been described as individuals whose virtues have become their vices (Malleson 2002). In their pre-fibromyalgia syndrome life they tend to have been highly motivated, overextended, self-critical, perfectionist and hardworking people who were, and remain, emotionally vulnerable tending to want to please others. They may or may not have realized how stressed they were but typically there were just not enough hours in the day to fit in all the things they needed to do. Very often their idea of recovery is to be able to achieve a state where they can actually do more than they were doing before they became ill, after all now they have to catch up. Needless to say for these individuals real relaxation skills and activity 'pacing' are nowhere on their agenda and are not easy for them to learn (Cedraschi et al 2004).

Frequently fibromyalgia syndrome patients, in common with a proportion of chronic fatigue syndrome patients and 'depressives', relate to others via a combination of putting others first and possibly 'emotional blackmail', sometimes in a context of catastrophizing (Hassett et al 2000).

The condition itself is defined via various diagnostic criteria (see Table 9.1). These generally recognized criteria appear specific and scientific but are the product of a committee process. Others identify fibromyalgia syndrome and chronic fatigue syndrome as the same condition (Wessely et al 1998) and some suggest connections between both of these conditions, thyroid dysfunction and/or 'gout'. The criteria are from the Copenhagen Declaration and represent 'medical opinion' rather than hard science. This combination of factors can make fibromyalgia syndrome patients challenging and exhausting to work with.

Since any realistic intervention programme has to deal with the whole person in their 'naturalistic' social setting it is a team game, but the therapist remains a key player. Despite the best plans and the best care it may be that success will be limited rather than absolute, about management and long-term coping skills rather than 'cure' (Nicassio et al 2000). Long-term coping skills can be affected by external factors such as casual statements or predictions by significant clinicians as the literature suggests. Case Study 9.1 explores the role of the therapist and the use of an approach based upon cognitive–behavioural principles, increasingly used in chronic medical problems (White 2001).

137

CASE STUDY 9.1

Patient profile

The person referred was a woman in her late forties, Mrs X, who had led a very busy life as a working mother and housewife. She had become ill nearly four years before during a period of marital problems. Because of severe pain, exhaustion and increasing debility Mrs X eventually had to use a wheelchair. Indeed from onset to the present it had been a story of increasing medication and decreasing health and functional ability. The marital problems became increasingly severe. Eventually (two years before her referral to physiotherapy) her husband had left her and was now living with a woman in her early thirties. Mrs X remained bitterly angry with her husband and considered that no matter how he felt he should have stayed with her to look after her and put her needs first after all the years when she had put his needs first. She had two sons, one of whom was temporarily living at home but was about to move in with his fiancée.

Approximately one year before her referral to physiotherapy in mental health a consultant had informed Mrs X that because of her (physical) medical condition she would have to use a wheelchair. On commencing physiotherapy she stated that she had just reconciled herself to this level of permanent disability and was beginning to organize her social life around being a permanent wheelchair user. Since being informed of the permanent nature of her disability by the consultant Mrs X had become very low in mood and her GP had referred her to mental health services where she had been informed that, as well as fibromyalgia syndrome, she had also developed depression. Despite her diagnosis of depression and the fibromyalgia syndrome there was no evidence of 'fibrofog' and Mrs X seemed able to remember everything clearly and talk eloquently and fulsomely, if sometimes emotionally, about all the issues around her condition.

Physically Mrs X was very weak, although she had normal ranges of movement with some pain. Mrs X could transfer well and easily but her assisted standing balance was poor. She stated that she was tender everywhere but was only noticeably tender and reacted to no more than six of the recognized tender points for fibromyalgia syndrome. Mrs X believed that she needed caring for by others, including Health and Social Services and her older son, the one at home. Previously an occupational therapist who had just left the NHS and who had also recently moved to another city had worked with her. The occupational therapist was now in private practice as an aromatherapist and had used this passive and very pleasant treatment modality with the patient, who had loved it, to alleviate symptoms.

Mrs X viewed herself as being a good mother who had worked until her illness and kept a spotless house.

- She had been a very sociable and outgoing person and although she was always full of fun she had always been a worrier, although not many people realized that.
- She had tried to do her best around everyone but now that she needed people where were they?
- She had to rely on people from Social Services whilst she waited for a cure, although she realized the latter was unlikely.
- She had always had a stressful life, even in her childhood. She had no siblings or close, surviving relatives in the area.
- She became ill easily from any cause, frequently having colds, upset stomachs and the like. Headaches were also an issue for her but she did not believe that they were stress headaches or that any of her problems were connected to stress of any kind in any way as that was a mental problem and her illnesses were completely physical.
- Her current hobby was writing, mainly about her illness, how she had suffered and how people had let her down. Recently she had started contacting other wheelchair users over the internet.

The assessment process

The initial assessment was conducted over three interviews, each incorporating some of the physical assessment. Motivational interviewing, described in Chapter 7 as 'a counselling style that facilitates an atmosphere of constructive conversation in which the health professional uses empathetic listening to gain insight into the client's perspective', was used to ascertain where the patient was in regard to the 'cycle of change' and what her beliefs (knowledge or cognitions) and behaviours were in relation to the fibromyalgia syndrome and how these affected her expectations (see Table 9.2 on page 141–142).

Secondly, an attempt was made to gauge her emotional reality and what characterized her relationships with others. Subsequently this was crosschecked with other members of the team. Thirdly and finally, the gentle physical assessment had two dimensions to it. The first was simple and purely physical, strength, range of movement, balance, pain/tender points etc. The second was to assess how her beliefs about her condition were being realized or expressed through the medium of body use and physical tension.

Beliefs can be characterized as helpful or unhelpful and it should be remembered, with reference to psychoneuroimmunological theory, that beliefs are realized via neurophysiological processes in terms of both neurotransmitters and neurohormones, the latter largely expressed via the neuroendocrine system, producing chemical and structural effects throughout the whole body. That is, a belief has a physical 'substance' in terms of its physiological expression and effects simply because any 'mental' process is made possible only by the 'hardware' of the nervous system and neuroendocrine system themselves indivisible in life from the rest of the body (see Chapter 3 for a full discussion); this has been explored principally in relation to pain (Haythornwaite et al 1998, Hyman 1999). This has been proposed as a model for the real, measurable, physiological changes produced by the 'placebo effect' and the 'nocebo effect'. In this context, the clinician should always strive to find a balance between honesty and maximizing the placebo effect (Klaber-Moffett & Richardson 1997).

This may be a difficult concept to grasp for patients and possibly some clinicians reared in a social environment where illnesses are either real and physical or psychological/psychosomatic and thus imagined according to a misinterpretation of Descartes (Kroenke & Swindle 2000, Moseley 2003). In the case of this patient the mind–body split had been combined with a nocebo effect to the extent that she had reinvented herself as the woman with the physical disability who would have to make the best of a life in a wheelchair. In terms of her mental health problems these had been simplified and stated in purely physical terms to the extent that almost precluded psychosocial intervention. The results of the assessment are outlined in the patient profile above and the problems that seemed to be salient from the assessment were:

- Negative beliefs regarding her prognosis (Jensen et al 2001).
- A belief that all her fibromyalgia syndrome-related problems were purely physical and unconnected to lifetime history of stress or to stress in any form.
- A belief that her depression was a separate disease and unconnected to her circumstances or history based upon a complete misconception of depression inculcated by professionals!
- A profound belief that any attempt to look at psychosocial factors indicated an absolute disbelief that her condition was 'real' and was an attempt to invalidate her suffering by identifying her problems as being 'all in my mind'.
- A belief that any reduction in symptoms would probably be restricted to reduction in pain by passive means.
- A belief that physical activity and exercise would exacerbate her problems.
- A belief that nutrition/diet or anything else that she could change herself was unlikely to affect her condition. (Her diet showed signs of type B malnutrition, adequate in calories but inadequate in nutrients.)
- Profound physical deconditioning that meant that any effort produced delayed onset muscle soreness and fatigue, misread as an increase in symptoms.
- Emotional lability characterized by rapid changes from bitter anger to self-pitying tears, sometimes both at the same time.

- A listing of most of the 'classic' traits and vulnerability factors for both fibromyalgia syndrome and depression including abuse, desertion and social isolation and 'performance' issues in the sense of playing a role of false confidence and self-immolation (Caspi et al 2003).

These were hardly 'predictors of success' (King et al 2002a).

From a cognitive–behavioural perspective, in the broad sense, the patient was living out the beliefs most likely to produce the predicted poor prognosis. Although she did have impairments largely resulting from fear-avoidance behaviour and deconditioning she had arrived at a point where her new 'authentic' self was aligned with the definitions provided by health-care professionals. In essence they had created a 'self-fulfilling prophesy', propelling her into disability (Martin et al 1996, Mengshoel & Haugen 2001).

Mrs X and the physiotherapist agreed on the range of needs (Table 9.3, p 142), and a 'menu' of possible interventions was created to meet her needs. The two key issues were reconditioning via a very gradual and progressive exercise programme and to use information to 'undercut' her current negative and disabling belief structure. However, these two issues could not be tackled head on. So a 'menu' was presented (Table 9.4, p 143), of different activities and these were discussed between Mrs X and the physiotherapist. Mrs X made the choice of starting with the massage. After three months of weekly massage, relaxation was introduced, along with the introduction of minimal exercise.

At around six months the physiotherapist discussed the central modulation concept of fibromyalgia syndrome taken from Crofford & Demitrack (1996) and Wessely et al (1998) with Mrs X. This explains how cortisol-related central nervous system changes, profoundly influenced by the neuroendocrine system and dependent on the reaction to stress produces the physiological changes, similar but ultimately unique in every case, that result in the subjective experience of fibromyalgia syndrome.

Following this explanation a significant development in treatment occurred using the stress/pain diary. Information on both perceived stress and perceived pain was collected in a tabular form by dividing the day in to three-hour blocks over a two-month period. In each block the patient provided a short statement about context and feelings and a numerical rating for stress and pain. Stress and pain were rated from 0 to 10. Very elegantly this revealed that an increase in stress was followed by an almost identically rated increase in pain with a one- to six-hour delay depending on the stressor. This conformed almost exactly to one of the predicted profiles and provided evidence to the patient that her condition was stress-related but realized via neurophysiological changes. This was the key factor in enabling a conceptual paradigm-shift and an increased internal locus of control.

After approximately nine months from referral the patient began to attend the physiotherapy department twice weekly for a programme that eventually grew to fifteen minutes on the exercise bike, up to forty minutes doing step-ups on a 'step aerobic' box on the highest level within the parallel bars and a forty- to sixty-minute weight-training programme followed by stretching and balance exercises. This was done in a group context and completely led by the technical instructor with up to twenty in- and out-patients of various ages passing through the gym during the same period. Some of these were 'individuals' seen by the attending physiotherapist.

After a further three months the physiotherapy staff discussed with Mrs X a move to attend a local leisure centre, supported by physiotherapy staff. Initially this involved one day attendance a week at the local leisure centre with the physiotherapist acting as a buddy and one day attendance at the physiotherapy gym.

In approximately eighteen months, and after more than four years of deterioration, the patient was able to come off antidepressants, although she required increased input and reassurance during the withdrawal phase. She had also greatly reduced her pain medication and had improved her diet. Although she could walk around the gym with little real assistance she refused to part with her wheelchair. Her new social life, persona or 'authentic' self and income were bound up with it.

From a physiotherapy perspective this case was successful with Mrs X maintaining herself at a functional level she could live with. Through help from other therapists including a community psychiatric nurse she had become more assertive and less critical and this had improved her relationships. Mrs X was now getting out of the house and was the prime mover in local wheelchair dancing. In reality she could probably have thrown away the wheelchair and improved well beyond these limitations but these were not her goals.

The system outlined above is based upon the care programme approach, amended in detail by the incorporation of motivational interviewing and a broad 'cognitive–behavioural' perspective. Cognitions and behaviours were both changed through the process. It will not always be successful in every case of fibromyalgia syndrome for a variety of reasons (Turk et al 1998, Van Houdenhove 2000). Cognitive–behavioural approaches provide a comprehensive, person-centred framework for addressing needs. The patient-selected interventions can be introduced at a rate appropriate to the individual; as such it provides a useful system for therapists.

Table 9.2 ● An outline of motivational interviewing

Principles	
Express empathy	Make it obvious that you are trying to understand their position, how they feel, what they know, how life is for them and all the issues that concern them
Avoid argumentation	Provide information in a neutral way that emphasizes that you respect their autonomy and their choices and that always leaves them in a position of feeling 'good' about themselves and positive about their working relationship with you
Roll with resistance	Always take into account 'readiness to change', as yet they may not be in a personal/social or psychological situation where they can contemplate change and resistance is indicative that you are trying to push the patient rather than putting them in a position of leading you in the direction that you want to go, towards change and improvement in their condition
Deploy discrepancy	Use ambivalence getting them to identify where they want to go and the beliefs and behaviours they have that prevent them. Provide information and support and ensure that the patient is the one who selects targets and ways forward from the OPTIONS
Support self-efficacy	The client has to be the active decision maker and has to be able to ensure that they do what they say that they will do. Look at barriers to change and identify what actions need to be taken to deal with and dismantle these barriers. Actively support change, especially in the initial stages

Table 9.2 ● Continued

Strategies		
Typical day		**Explore concerns**
Negotiating a plan		Consider all the options
Readiness to change/confidence they can change (self-efficacy)		Arrive at a plan
Good and not so good results of change		Costs/benefits analysis
Looking back		Looking forward
Tactics/micro-skills		
Open-ended questions		Reflective listening
Affirmations		Summaries

Table 9.3 ● List of needs generated via negotiation and agreed with the patient

1. A reduction of perceived pain
2. An improvement of general well-being and health. (This would include nutrition)
3. An increased understanding of the wider information and research or evidence in relation to FMS and depression
4. A gradual improvement of physical functional ability in as much as this would be possible
5. An improvement in mood and reduction of emotional lability
6. Improved relationships with people currently in her life so that she felt supported and did not feel exploited
7. Getting out of the house more and building an actual social life rather than a virtual one via the internet. (Currently focused on making contacts with wheelchair users who were also largely disabled by their environment and/or the people around them)
8. To have treats, something entirely for herself that would be indulgent but good for her health and/or well-being in some way

Table 9.4 ● Possible interventions to meet the listed needs

Needs met	Possible interventions

(a) Massage. Since aromatherapy had been used before the physiotherapist suggested using something similarly alternative, namely Shiatsu-based massage after explanations of its possible effects (e.g. increasing oxytocin, human growth factor, serotonin and dopamine, decreases of cortisol, adrenaline, noradrenaline, possible disinhibition of the opiate-peptide system and the effects this might have on adult neurogenesis, synaptic connections and other neurochemicals such as GABA). This led to explaining how exercise could have some similar effects and, in particular, could affect GABA-ergic pathways originating in the cerebellum. The physiotherapist explained the possible implications of this in relation to pain, healing, and states of mind including affect

(b) Relaxation. Ideally the physiotherapist would have used deep relaxation, really more or less indistinguishable from hypnosis, with a tailored 'covert rehearsal' as this has been used to reduce pain and improve physical performance. However Mrs X found this impossible. Mrs X settled on autogenic training with a spoken script (Keel at al 1998, Rossi & Cheek 1994)

(c) Body awareness via postural exercises and 'dynamic relaxation' techniques. These sessions included discussion on the psychological impact of exercise regarding internal locus of control and self-efficacy, self-esteem and self-concept. The focus was on getting the patient to 'listen' to her own body and act on what she 'heard', to embrace pacing and regularly change her activities without over-stretching herself physically

(d) Referral to a dietitian for nutritional input to use food as a form of chemical intervention. The patient kept a diary of her diet for two weeks and the dietitian compared this to optimum nutritional needs identified in the literature

(e) Referral to occupational therapist to look at 'activity' in and out of the home, from dressing to hobbies to occupation

(f) A progressive exercise regimer to eventually include resistance training (King et al 2002b, Gowans et al 2001, Taylor 2000, Jones et al 2002)

(g) An information programme. The physiotherapist also helped with the initial access to websites and provided handouts and leaflets, including a large selection from the local library and community centre regarding activities

(h) Support into making use of local activities for local people with disabilities. (Eventually the patient helped to organize a wheelchair-dancing club in the area – there were pros and cons to this in the long term)

(i) Day trips out

(j) Support into other social contacts and around personal relationships

(k) Keeping a task-related diary. Diary 1 was a listing of her diet. Diary 2 was a listing of perceived stress and perceived pain

143

Key Messages

- Fibromyalgia syndrome is a heterogeneous chronic pain condition that is thought to be stress related.
- The diagnostic criteria for fibromyalgia syndrome include widespread unexplained pain with the presence of multiple tender points.
- Cognitive–behavioural approaches can be used successfully with some people in the management of fibromyalgia syndrome but the evidence base is limited.
- Motivational interviewing used within a cognitive–behavioural approach is a useful technique to establish the patient's perspective and can be utilized within the physiotherapy and occupational therapy assessment.

References

Carli G, Suman A L, Badii F et al 2000 Differences between patients with fibromyalgia and patients with chronic musculoskeletal pain. In: Devor M, Rowbotham M C, Wiesenfeld-Hallin Z (eds) Proceedings of the 9th World Congress on Pain. Progress in Pain Research and Management 16(97): 1031–1037. IASP Press, Seattle, WA

Caspi A, Sugden K, Moffitt T E et al 2003 Influence of life stress on depression: moderation by a polymorphism in the 5-HTT gene. Science 18:301(5631):291–293

Cedraschi C, Desmeules J, Rapiti E et al 2004 Fibromyalgia: a randomised, controlled trial for a treatment programme based on self-management. Annals of Rheumatic Disease 63(3):290–296

Clauw D J, Crofford L J 2003 Chronic widespread pain and fibromyalgia: what we know, and what we need to know. Best Practice Research in Clinical Rheumatology 17(4):685–701

Crofford L J, Demitrack M A 1996 Evidence that abnormalities of central neurohormonal systems are key to understanding fibromyalgia and chronic fatigue syndrome. Rheumatic Disease Clinics of North America 22(2):267–284

Earnshaw S M, MacGregor G, Dawson JK 2001 Fibromyalgia – monotheories, monotherapies and reductionism. Rheumatology 40:348–349

Gowans S E, deHueck A, Voss S et al 2001 Effect of a randomized, controlled trial of exercise on mood and physical function in individuals with fibromyalgia. Arthritis and Rheumatism 45(6):519–529

Hadler N M 1997 Fibromyalgia, chronic fatigue, and other iatrogenic diagnostic algorithms: do some labels escalate illness in vulnerable patients? Postgraduate Medicine 102(2):161–177

Hassett A L, Cone J D, Patella S J et al 2000 The role of catastrophizing in the pain and depression of women with fibromyalgia syndrome. Arthritis and Rheumatism 43(11):2493–2500

Haythornwaite J A, Menefee L A, Heinberg L J et al 1998 Pain coping strategies predict perceived control over pain. Pain 77(1): 33–39

Hazemeijer I, Rasker J J 2003 A review of fibromyalgia and related syndromes. Rheumatology 42:507–515

Hyman R 1999 The mischief-making of ideomotor action. The Scientific Review of Alternative Medicine 3(2):34–43

Jensen M P, Turner J A, Romano J M 2001 Changes in beliefs, catastrophizing, and coping are associated with improvement in multidisciplinary pain treatment. Journal of Consultative Clinical Psychology 69(4):655–662

Jones K D, Burckhardt C S, Clark S R et al 2002 A randomized controlled trial of muscle strengthening versus flexibility training in fibromyalgia. The Journal of Rheumatology 29(5):1041–1048

Keel P J, Bodoky C, Gerhard U et al 1998 Comparison of group therapy and group relaxation training for fibromyalgia. Clinical Journal of Pain 14(3):232–238

King S J, Wessel J, Bhambhani Y et al 2002a Predictors of success of intervention programmes for persons with fibromyalgia. Journal of Rheumatology 29(5):1034–1040

King S J, Wessel J, Bhambhani Y et al 2002b The effects of exercise and education, individually or combined, in women with fibromyalgia. Journal of Rheumatology 29(12):2620–2627

Klaber-Moffett J, Richardson P 1997 The influence of the physiotherapist–patient relationship on pain and disability. Physiotherapy Theory and Practice 11:3–11

Kroenke K, Swindle R 2000 Cognitive-behavioural therapy for somatization and symptom syndromes: a critical review of controlled clinical trials. Psychotherapeutic Psychosomatics 69(4):205–215

Malleson A 2002 Whiplash and other useful illnesses. McGill-Queen's University Press (2003 reprint)

Martin M Y, Bradley L A, Alexander R W et al 1996 Coping strategies predict disabilities in patients with primary fibromyalgia. Pain 68(1):45–53

Mengshoel A M, Haugen M 2001 Health status in fibromyalgia – a follow up study. Journal of Rheumatology 45(4):355–361

Moseley L 2003 Unravelling the barriers to reconceptualization of the problem in chronic pain: the actual and perceived ability of patients and health professionals to understand the neurophysiology. Journal of Pain 4(4):184–189

Nicassio P M, Weisman M H, Schumann C et al 2000 The role of generalized pain and pain behaviour in tender point scores in fibromyalgia. Journal of Rheumatology 27(4):1056–1062

Raphael K G, Janal M N, Nayak S et al 2004 Familial aggregation of depression in fibromyalgia: a community based test of alternate hypotheses. Pain 110(1–2):449–460 Comment in Pain 2004 112(3):409–410; author reply 410

Rossi E L, Cheek D B 1994 Mind–body therapy methods of ideodynamic healing in hypnosis. W W Norton, London, pp 9–34, 238–259

Sherman J J, Turk D C, Okifuji A 2000 Prevalence and impact of post-traumatic stress disorder-like symptoms on patients with fibromyalgia syndrome. Clinical Journal of Pain 16:127–134

Starlanyl P J, Copeland M E 1996 Fibromyalgia and chronic myofascial pain syndrome: a survival manual. New Harbinger Publications, Oakland, CA

Taylor A 2000 Physical activity, anxiety and stress. In: Biddle S J H, Fox K R, Boutcher S H (eds) Physical activity and psychological well-being. Routledge, London, pp 10–45

Turk D C, Okifuji A Sinclair J D et al 1998 Differential responses by psychosocial subgroups of fibromyalgia syndrome patients to an interdisciplinary treatment. Arthritis Care Research 11(5):397–404

Van Houdenhove B 2000 Psychosocial stress and chronic pain. European Journal of Pain 4:225–228

Wessely S, Hotopf M, Sharpe M 1998 Chronic fatigue and its syndromes. Oxford University Press, Oxford, pp 250–276

White C A 2001 Cognitive behaviour therapy for chronic medical problems a guide to assessment and treatment in practice. John Wiley, Chichester, pp 4–35, 60, 123–147

Chronic fatigue syndrome

Tina Everett and Anne Stewart

10

Introduction

Chronic fatigue syndrome (CFS) is defined in its historical and community context with reference to self-help groups and internet information. The evidence for cognitive–behavioural therapy (CBT) and other interventions is reviewed and a rationale given for a cognitive whole-team approach to graded exercise and recovery. The cognitive model for the assessment of CFS and illness beliefs is discussed and a plan of intervention is outlined, with a case example of an adolescent with CFS.

Chronic fatigue was recognized formally as a medical condition around the middle of the nineteenth century (Wessely et al 1998). The term ME (myalgic encephalomyelitis) was first used in the 1970s and was widely adopted by support groups such as the ME Association. The term CFS has been widely accepted in health care since the early 1990s, although the large majority of patient support organizations continue to use the term ME. The Independent Working Group (2002) used the composite term CFS/ME, acknowledging that neither term is entirely acceptable to both patients and clinicians. The prevalence of CFS/ME in the UK ranges from 0.4% to 2.6%, according to different studies (Gallagher et al 2004). A general practice with 10,000 patients is likely to have 30–40 patients with CFS/ME (Price & Couper 2003).

Research initially focused largely on the cause and pathology of CFS (Pemberton et al 1994) and less on rehabilitation. Since the late 1990s there has been more emphasis on intervention, and the evidence base of CBT in chronic fatigue has been researched, including a Cochrane Review (Clements et al 1997, Price & Couper 1999, 2003).

Seven different categories of intervention have been evaluated in the Cochrane review for their potential use in the management of CFS/ME: behavioural, immunological, antiviral, pharmacological, supplements, complementary/alternative and multitreatment. Interventions which have been studied using randomized controlled trials include CBT and graded exercise therapy (Price & Couper 2003).

Clinical description

Patients with chronic fatigue describe feelings of exhaustion, often exacerbated by minor activity and requiring marked reduction in activity or even confinement to bed in severe cases. Sufferers frequently report other symptoms such as headaches, sleeping difficulties, muscle aching, sore throats, tender lymph nodes, and cognitive symptoms such as poor memory and concentration.

Research into comorbidity suggests that approximately 50% of young people and 40–70% of adults seen in specialist services have a psychiatric disorder when their chronic fatigue is diagnosed, particularly depression or anxiety (Garralda et al 1999, Wessely et al 1998).

Diagnosis

There is no specific constellation of symptoms or laboratory test that identifies the presence of chronic fatigue and, as fatigue is a common symptom in the community, choosing the cut-off point for CFS is inevitably somewhat arbitrary. However, there are two groups who have developed criteria for diagnosis, whilst acknowledging the dimensional nature to the condition.

The 1995 Oxford consensus meeting agreed to establish a set of diagnostic criteria for CFS and they have become known as the Oxford criteria, defined as:

- At least six months duration
- Definite onset
- Impaired function (in activities of daily living and/or social engagement)
- Physical and mental fatigability
- Myalgia
- Mood and sleep disturbance.

The exclusion criteria are:

- Extensive list of physical causes
- Psychosis
- Bipolar disorder
- Substance abuse.

A history of psychiatric illness (apart from the above criteria) does not come into the Oxford exclusion criteria for diagnosis.

The other group that has developed criteria is the Centre for Disease Control, USA (see Box 10.1). The CDC criteria place a greater emphasis on physical symptoms and also exclude severe depression (Fukuda et al 1994). Both sets of criteria are frequently used in research studies.

Ideally, it is best to delay treatment until physical investigations are complete and a definite diagnosis of chronic fatigue has been given.

Young people

Reports have indicated that CFS is less common in children than adults (Jordan et al 1998, Gallagher et al 2004). Chalder et al (2003) found that symptomatic fatigue in

> ## Box 10.1
>
> ### CDC criteria (Fukuda et al 1994)
>
> #### Major criteria
>
> - Debilitating fatigue reducing activity to less than 50% of the patient's premorbid activity for at least six months
> - Symptoms not explained by other medical or chronic psychiatric illness
>
>   The presence of non-psychotic depression does not preclude the diagnosis of chronic fatigue syndrome
>
> #### Symptom criteria (four required)
>
> - Sore throat
> - Painful cervical or axillary lymphadenopathy
> - Muscle discomfort or pain
> - Prolonged generalized fatigue after usual levels of activity
> - Headaches
> - Arthralgia (without swelling or redness)
> - Neuropsychological disorders such as forgetfulness and lack of concentration
> - Sleep disturbance (unrefreshing sleep)

children is common; however, chronic fatigue and CFS are relatively rare. Reporting of somatic symptoms, including fatigue, increases during adolescence and early adulthood (Eminson et al 1996). Most children with CFS also have impaired school attendance or performance and a decrease in social activities (Carter et al 1995). It has been suggested that CFS is the commonest current cause of long-term school non-attendance (Wright et al 1999). Garralda (1999) recommends reducing the six-month duration criteria to three months for diagnosis of children and adolescents, to allow earlier recognition and to reduce the risk of long-term school absenteeism with prolonged disability.

Evidence base for treatment and outcome

Chronic fatigue is a disorder involving physical symptoms, psychological distress and unhelpful beliefs about the disorder. Afari & Buchwald (2003) found that people with CFS often attribute their illness to physical causes and minimize psychological and personal contributions. However, Wessely et al (1998) suggests that in terms of treatment outcome it is not the beliefs about causes which are important, rather the beliefs about maintaining factors such as activity, exercise and rest. Research has focused both on physical rehabilitation and the use of CBT to address unhelpful thoughts and beliefs.

The most recent Cochrane review of CBT (Price & Couper 1999, 2003) systematically reviewed randomized controlled trials of CBT for adults with CFS. They tested the hypothesis that CBT is more effective than orthodox medical management or other interventions for adults with CFS. Only three relevant trials of adequate quality were found (Sharpe et al 1996, Deale et al 1997, Lloyd et al 1993) and these all demonstrated that CBT significantly benefits physical functioning in adult out-patients with CFS when compared to orthodox medical management or relaxation. Other reviewers substantiate the Cochrane review (Whiting et al 2002). However, a study by Deale et al (2001) on long-term outcomes of CBT states that once therapy ends some people have difficulty making further improvements. They recommend that attention be given to maintaining and extending gains after regular treatment ends. Follow-up sessions are likely to have an important role in helping to maintain improvements.

Graded exercise was advocated by Fulcher & White (1998); they recommend a graded increase in activity but with full cooperation of the individual, and opportunity given for slowing the pace or remaining static if symptoms increase. A later audit on the success of this treatment regimen concluded that graded exercise therapy should be more widely available in general physiotherapy departments by specially trained therapists (White & Naish 2001). A recent study of patient education to encourage graded exercise in CFS demonstrated that a cognitive approach may be as effective as formal CBT but is shorter and requires less therapist skill (Powell et al 2001).

With regard to the younger age group, Chalder et al (2002) has found that family-focused CBT was effective in improving functioning and reducing fatigue in 11–18-year-olds. A limitation of this study was that it lacked a control group. A randomized controlled study has now been carried out and the results are awaited.

Regarding outcome, a systematic review found that 54–94% of children make a good recovery (Joyce et al 1997). Good outcome is related to having a specific physical trigger, the start of the illness in the autumn term and higher socio-economic status (Rangel et al 2000a). Garralda & Rangel (2001) reported that beliefs about the presence of physical illness in the young person and their parents were associated with poorer outcome. However, the numbers in this study were small.

In adults, prognosis is less good, particularly those seen in specialist settings. Fewer than 10% of CFS patients referred to specialist settings make a full recovery (Wilson et al 1994). A number of poor prognostic factors have been reported, including older age, chronicity, comorbid psychiatric disorder, holding a belief that the illness is due to physical causes (Joyce et al 1997) and being a member of a self-help organization (Sharpe et al 1992). An association between degree of impairment and a passive coping strategy has also been described (Deale et al 1998, Ray et al 1995).

In summary, the evidence to date suggests that a combination of graded exercise and a cognitive approach can be helpful in the treatment of chronic fatigue. Occu-pational therapists (OTs) and physiotherapists (PTs) can make a useful contribution to treatment of both mild and more severe cases, as described later.

Sources of information accessible to patients

Patients with CFS and their families now have access to many sources of infor-mation, not all of which are consistent, particularly regarding the role of activity and rest. These sources include: the internet, self-help groups, advice from sports instructors, self-help books, schools, and also health professionals. These are described in more detail at the end of this chapter.

Integrating CBT within physiotherapy and occupational therapy

Evidence suggests that incorporating a cognitive approach in the physical management of chronic fatigue can be beneficial. Patients with chronic fatigue are frequently referred to physiotherapists (PTs) and occupational therapists (OTs) for assessment and management, either direct from primary care, or as part of a specialist team. There is evidence that the shorter the duration of illness before treatment the better the prognosis (Wessely et al 1998), making early intervention crucial for this condition. PTs and OTs may be involved at an early stage of treatment. Ideally, they work as part of a specialist team, but the community therapist, working in isolation will also find the 'Treatment Techniques' section of this chapter of benefit, provided they can refer to a psychology service if symptoms persist.

An understanding of the cognitive, emotional and behavioural aspects that contribute to the development and maintenance of chronic fatigue is essential in working with people with CFS. Illness beliefs may impact significantly on the patient's ability to use the strategies recommended by therapists, and these beliefs need to be addressed directly to facilitate recovery (see Case Study 10.1 on page 158–160). For more severe cases a joint approach between psychiatrist, psychologist and psychiatric nurse and PT/OTs can be productive, with each professional addressing psychological factors using their particular skills and emphasis. With a joint approach it is still essential for PTs and OTs to be able to work with belief systems in order to motivate patients and help them progress. Training in the use of cognitive–behavioural techniques for all professions is thus very relevant.

Cognitive model of chronic fatigue

There is no established single cause for chronic fatigue syndrome. Research has identified a range of factors contributing to both the development and the maintenance of chronic fatigue. However, the evidence to date is limited. A cognitive–behavioural model has been proposed in order to understand the development and maintenance of the disorder (David et al 1991, Wessely et al 1998). The following model incorporates ideas from Wessely's model and takes account of factors identified by research.

Predisposing factors

Organic factors may predispose to the development of chronic fatigue in some cases. The hypothalamic–pituitary–adrenal axis component of the hormonal stress response has been examined in patients with CFS, indicating the possibility of dysregulation in some patients, giving rise to vulnerability (Cleare & Wessely 1996).

Psychological factors, including temperament and coping styles, can also predispose an individual to developing CFS. Rangel et al (2000b) found that adolescents with chronic fatigue were more likely to be sensitive, conforming and dependent, with a tendency towards obsessive or perfectionistic personality traits. These young people may show underlying low self-esteem, with core beliefs such as: 'I am vulnerable', 'I am worthless'. These core beliefs can lead to dysfunctional assumptions such as 'I must perform to a high standard to be accepted'. Typical personality features in people who develop chronic fatigue are the need to strive for high standards, and a tendency towards rigidity and anxiety (Rangel et al 2000b).

Triggers

Fatigue may be triggered by a number of factors, such as a virus infection (including glandular fever) (Rangel et al 2000b), or a stressful life event (Theorell et al 1999); these can lead to a reduced ability to meet demands, poor sleeping and loss of energy. In young people, transferring to a new school can be a stressful event which triggers the condition. The direct effect of a virus illness on muscles is also relevant to the emergence of fatigue symptoms. The advice given at this stage by family and by professionals may be crucial in determining whether a person develops either helpful illness beliefs, leading to graded exercise and a reduction of stress, or alternatively unhelpful illness beliefs, which may lead to prolonged periods of rest or continued excessive activity, which in turn may lead to chronic fatigue syndrome.

Maintenance

Once fatigue has developed, a number of factors may maintain it (see Figure 10.1). Wessely et al (1998) has characterized the behavioural responses to fatigue and Fulcher & White (1997) describe the notion of 'physical deconditioning', which refers to the widespread effects of physical inactivity.

When fatigued, the person may believe that the best course of action is to rest; if this rest is prolonged, the result is physical deconditioning with further muscle fatigue and muscle pain on resumption of activity. Fear of an exacerbation of symptoms can lead to increased inactivity and further effects of deconditioning. Alternatively, the drive to get better quickly can lead to excessive activity and ensuing overtiredness, necessitating further periods of rest. Difficulties in sleeping can exacerbate the daytime fatigue. Lack of progress can lead to feelings of demoralization and frustration, causing further reduction of activity, or bursts of overactivity. The sufferer may become overfocused on physical symptoms in an effort to address their problem and this preoccupation can also maintain the experience of fatigue (Ray et al 1995). Excessive reassurance seeking from family, friends or professionals can reinforce the unhelpful beliefs and result in heightened anxiety, which may contribute to further inactivity.

Consequences of prolonged inactivity, including loss of confidence socially, gradual withdrawal from friends, loss of muscle strength and decreased self-efficacy, can contribute to increased low mood or anxiety, both of which makes it harder to tackle the problems. Prolonged absence from work or school can lead to loss of confidence and anxiety about returning to normal routines.

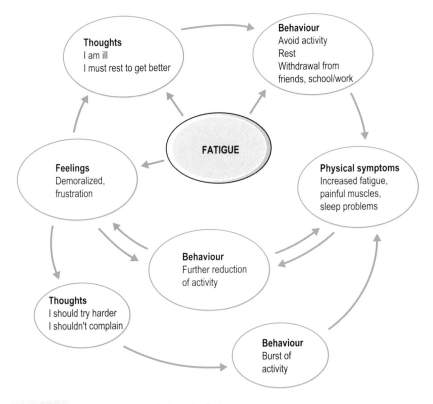

Figure 10.1 • Maintenance of chronic fatigue.

153

The cognitive–behavioural intervention is based on this model. Maintaining factors are addressed initially, and later in the therapy other issues, such as perfectionism, or low self-esteem, may be addressed. The main aim of treatment is to facilitate patients, supported by partner or family, in carrying out their own rehabilitation programme.

Treatment techniques

Assessment and engagement

A comprehensive assessment is the first step. This should include a history of the development of the problems and a detailed description of the current symptoms.

Alongside this description, a behavioural analysis of exactly what the person is able to do is essential. Asking the person to keep a diary, indicating activity, rest and sleep patterns helps to clarify what is happening. In order to give as accurate a picture as possible the diary should be filled in at the time that things happen. This diary can also be used as a way of monitoring progress over the course of treatment

Day and Date..

Number of hours sleep:

7.00 am	5.00 pm
8.00 am	6.00 pm
9.00 am	7.00 pm
10.00 am	8.00 pm
11.00 am	9.00 pm
12.00 pm	10.00 pm
1.00 pm	11.00 pm
2.00 pm	12.00 am
3.00 pm	
4.00 pm	

Comments on how the day went

_____

_____

_____

_____

_____

Figure 10.2 Daily activity and sleep record.

(see Figure 10.2 for an example of a diary). An exploration of factors relevant to the development of the chronic fatigue provides helpful information that can be used in producing the formulation and explaining the rationale for treatment. It is useful to identify coping strategies which have already been tried, and the outcome of these strategies. If there has been previous treatment for chronic fatigue it is useful to clarify the response to this treatment in order to avoid repeating unhelpful strategies. The patient should be asked explicitly what has helped or what has hindered progress in the past.

Discussion with parents/carers/partners can also be extremely helpful at this stage.

It is also important in the assessment to check for the presence of depression or anxiety, as these disorders may need additional treatment by psychiatrists or psychologists.

Establishing a good rapport is essential. Time taken to get to know the person, their interests, occupation, social relationships and usual way of responding to events, is well spent as it makes it clear to the patient that the therapist is interested in them as a whole person. It is important to convey a belief in the reality of the symptoms and a desire to understand more about the person's experience. It is not helpful to engage in discussion about whether the cause is physical or psychological, but instead to look at factors that can promote recovery, including behavioural, physical, emotional and cognitive factors. This may include discussing how a wide range of factors can contribute to progress, including improving sleep patterns, eating, motivation, addressing low mood and anxiety as well as actively addressing the symptoms of fatigue. During the assessment, it is helpful to acknowledge that this is a serious illness, which can lead to a number of adverse consequences. It is important to explain to the patient the numerous physical effects of deconditioning, such as decreased muscle strength, decreased aerobic capacity, decreased blood pressure, increased resting heart rate, all of which can contribute to increase in fatigue symptoms. It is also important to explain that graded exercise, together with a cognitive approach, is the treatment of choice and to acknowledge that the person with CFS may have mixed feelings about the process of treatment.

Cognitive formulation

As the assessment proceeds, information will be collected that can be used to build up an individual patient formulation, based on the cognitive model described earlier. It is important to develop this collaboratively, using Socratic questioning and guided discovery (see Appendix). A joint formulation, particularly focusing on maintenance factors, is the cornerstone of treatment, and leads logically to appropriate management approaches. The person is more likely to understand and agree with the rationale for treatment if they are involved closely in building up a comprehensive understanding of their problems. Key features to be included in the formulation are the cycles of inactivity and overactivity, both of which can contribute to muscle pain, weakness and worsening of the fatigue (see Figure 10.1). Completing the formulation provides a good opportunity to discuss with the patient the physical effects of rest as described earlier.

The initial collaborative formulation will shape the structure and focus of treatment. Treatment sessions should be regular, ideally once a week initially, moving to fortnightly as engagement becomes established. The focus on gradual, paced increases in activity needs to be fully explained, giving the person opportunity to discuss any difficulties or any thoughts/beliefs that might interfere with this programme.

Initial phase of treatment

The initial stage of treatment involves setting up realistic and achievable behavioural targets for each day. Scheduled rest periods must be built in, so that the person can develop a regular routine that includes a balance of rest and activity, planned in advance. The links between experiencing symptoms of fatigue and resting need to be gradually weakened. Some people prefer to have structured advice on specific exercises that can help to build up strength in a graded way, while others find that more functional activities, developed gradually, help to break the boom-and-bust cycles. It is important to continue to monitor daily activities so that progress can be tracked and facilitated (see Table 10.1).

Table 10.1 ● Positive data log

Old belief: I have to do everything perfectly otherwise people won't like me New belief: People will still like me even if I don't do everything perfectly			
Day	**Time**	**Situation**	**Evidence to support new belief**
Tues	6pm	Forgot to ring my friend when I said I was going to	My friend rang me later and we had a good chat. She was OK about me forgetting
Wed	12pm	Got my marks back from my Geography project Had not spent all night on it as I usually do	Marks were a bit lower than usual but my teacher still thinks I am good at Geography and I had time for other things too
Sat	2pm	Made a cake for my friend's birthday	It didn't turn out very well, but she was very pleased that I had made the effort and it didn't matter that it wasn't perfect

Strategies need to be introduced to improve sleeping patterns. Developing a routine of going to bed and getting up at structured times, whilst at the same time reducing sleep during the day, can be helpful in addressing sleeping difficulties.

As treatment proceeds, it is common for unhelpful thoughts or beliefs to get in the way of progress. For instance, the person may hold a belief about the harmful effects of exercise and the need to rest as a way of promoting recovery. It can be helpful to record these thoughts and develop ways of challenging them (see Table 4.4 on page 70 for an example of challenging negative automatic thoughts). Referring back to the formulation can help with this process. Setting up behavioural experiments to test unhelpful thoughts can also be productive, for example: monitoring the fatigue levels following a prolonged period of inactivity and a period of paced activity.

In addition it is helpful to develop a problem-solving approach to deal with physical symptoms such as headaches, or feeling unwell, or increased fatigue. Symptoms of anxiety or depression are common during the course of treatment. Those with severe depression may benefit from antidepressant treatment, although in others mood may improve with an increase in activity and social engagement. Where there is severe depression, it may be helpful to refer on to a psychologist for specific CBT for depression (see Chapter 4). With regard to anxiety, discussion of the physiological symptoms of anxiety can be helpful, along with anxiety management techniques and the role of safety behaviours (see Chapter 5).

Middle phase of treatment

By this stage, the person has developed strategies for coping with fatigue and is becoming more active. However, psychosocial problems may now emerge, such as relationship difficulties or issues related to return to work or school (see Case Study 10.1). The person may reach a plateau and find it difficult to progress to the next stage. Further unhelpful thoughts may become apparent, such as 'Will I ever get back to work? Am I going to get ill again?' These thoughts can be addressed systematically, encouraging a problem-solving approach and helping the person to develop more helpful thoughts.

People with chronic fatigue are often low in self-esteem. At this stage in treatment, underlying core beliefs such as: 'I am no good', 'No-one likes me' or dysfunctional assumptions such as 'I have to do everything perfectly for people to like me', may need to be addressed. Strategies include reviewing the evidence for and against the beliefs, exploring the effect of holding the belief and then building up an alternative belief. Beginning to collect evidence for the new belief (Table 10.1) can help the person start to notice signs which are consistent with the new belief, and which may have been ignored previously (Padesky 1994). The aim is to help the person feel better about him/herself and build confidence. During this phase, there needs to be continued work on gradually increasing activity.

Final phase (relapse prevention)

In the later stages of treatment relapse prevention is important. Setbacks can be predicted and coping strategies to cope with setbacks discussed in advance. Any remaining steps to achieve change should be explored, and it is helpful to collaborate with the person to produce a summary of progress. A phased follow-up can be helpful with reviews at increasing time intervals.

Working with young people and families

In working with young people it is important to consider the role of the family, both in the formulation of the problems and in the way family members can contribute to treatment (see Case Study 10.1). It is important to involve the parents from the start in helping to build up an understanding of their child's symptoms. Parents' beliefs about activity, rest or exercise should be explored in relation to their child's illness. Parents may feel guilty about encouraging their child to do more when this results in increased symptoms in the short term. Parents will, therefore, need to be helped to support their child's treatment plan. Ideally, once the parents are fully involved they can act as co-therapists, providing extra support at home to help their child challenge beliefs and progress through the programme. The formulation can be simplified in an appropriate way to make it easily understood by a younger child; however, the principles remain the same.

Liaison with schools

Return to school can be daunting, particularly if there has been a long period of absence, with loss of confidence and withdrawal from social relationships. Considerable encouragement and support will be needed to re-establish full-time education.

Schools usually play an important role in the progress of a young person with chronic fatigue. It may be helpful to initiate a meeting with their school in order to agree how best to provide support. It is important that school staff understand the reality of the physical symptoms, while at the same time realizing the need for gradual, paced activity. It can be helpful to reduce the number of examinations being undertaken.

In some circumstances, an explanation to other pupils can also be helpful. One adolescent designed a leaflet for other pupils in her class, explaining the symptoms of chronic fatigue in order to help them understand why she needed to take so much time off school. This proved a helpful way of enlisting the support and help of her classmates.

CASE STUDY 10.1

Sophie, aged 16, was referred to a child and adolescent clinic with long-term symptoms of fatigue. Following a positive test for glandular fever a year previously, she remained unwell, with enlarged glands and symptoms of fatigue. Although she initially returned to school, her attendance gradually dropped off and she spent increasing amounts of time at home, rarely going out. She found it hard to concentrate on school work, consequently got behind with her work and was anxious about returning to school. Her friends gradually stopped visiting her and she became isolated and low in mood. She began to find bright lights or loud sounds difficult to tolerate and increasingly shut herself off in her darkened bedroom. Her parents supported her as best they could; they were understandably concerned about underlying physical illness and worked hard to care for her physical needs and protect her from further stress. A medical assessment confirmed the diagnosis of CFS.

Sophie's early development was entirely normal. She was described as a very kind, caring and sociable person who was academically gifted and a high achiever. She had become ill in her GCSE year and subsequently did not sit her GCSEs. This was an enormous blow to her self-esteem as she had been predicted excellent grades. Her father was a managing director, with perfectionist traits and a tendency to work long hours; her mother was a teacher at a secondary school, also very committed to her work. A number of family members had recently had serious physical illness: paternal grandfather had died from cancer a year previously, and maternal grandmother died from cancer, after a long illness, six months later.

Sophie acknowledged frustration at her situation but at the same time found it difficult to make changes. She was fearful of doing too much in case her symptoms became worse. She realized that she needed help, but was very anxious about the sort of help she may receive. She agreed to see a physiotherapist and a psychologist and engage in a graded exercise programme alongside a CBT approach. The family, also, were keen to be involved, although initially sceptical that this approach could help.

The first step was to draw up a list of her problems and goals before creating together a simple formulation of her problems. Sophie began to work out the things that were maintaining and exacerbating her problems; however, she was afraid of making changes and found it hard to keep to her exercise schedule. The physiotherapist worked out with her a plan of exercises to build up muscle strength and functional tasks to help break the vicious cycles. She was able to see that negative thoughts such as: 'It's no good, I am never going to get better', 'I must stop as soon as I feel a twinge of fatigue' were holding her back. In her sessions with the psychologist, she began to challenge these thoughts, learning to replace them with more realistic and helpful thoughts. These changes in thinking were also reinforced in her sessions with the physiotherapist (PT). In exercising with the physiotherapist Sophie was pleased to find her stamina slowly improving. The PT asked her to write down any thoughts she had before, during or after her daily exercise schedule. The PT was able to encourage positive feelings, and when negative thoughts were expressed she would remind Sophie of her work with the psychologist and ask her to come up with a more positive alternative. When Sophie complained of muscle aches and pains during or after exercise the PT would give a physical explanation and specific postural exercises and advice. These strategies were then reinforced in the family meeting.

Sophie's parents remained concerned and wanted further physical investigations to exclude other physical causes. They still believed that Sophie had a serious physical illness. However, the paediatrician was confident that further investigations were not necessary. Sophie's parents were encouraged to develop a more helpful appraisal of her illness and what could be done about it. They were helped to focus more on what was maintaining the problem, particularly the inactivity, rather than trying to find out and being preoccupied with the cause.

Sophie kept a record of her activity, sleep patterns, thoughts and feelings and was able to see changes over time. Eventually she was able to go out of the house and plucked up courage to contact a friend and arrange a meeting. The positive feelings that arose from this meeting gave her the courage to try further social activities and she began to build up confidence. She was extremely anxious at the thought of returning to school and after discussions with relevant professionals arranged to finish her GCSEs, studying part time at a local college. A meeting was held with her college tutor to plan a gradual integration into college. She began to attend one morning a week initially, gradually increasing her hours. Sophie found resuming her studies very difficult and scary, but was helped by the occupational therapist who used a problem-solving approach, with focused targets, positive reinforcement and challenge of negativity.

Four months into treatment Sophie had a major relapse following a throat infection. She retired to bed and found it difficult to mobilize herself again. The reality of her physical symptoms was acknowledged and a plan of action was drawn up with graded exercise. She drew on the skills she had already learnt and managed to avoid getting caught up in the vicious cycles of rest and bursts of activity, as she might have done previously. She was more easily able to resume her studies at college.

Towards the end of treatment a review meeting was held involving Sophie, her parents and the treatment team. Sophie was encouraged in advance to draw up her summary of progress.

The summary was drawn up using the following key questions:

1. How did my problem develop?

    I had glandular fever which made me very tired. When I went back to school I found it hard to keep up with the work. I began to miss school more and more and stayed at home as I felt so tired.

2. What kept it going?

    At home I was sitting around doing nothing and my muscles just got weaker.
    I felt guilty and would go for a walk but I overdid it and felt worse.
    I didn't really feel like eating and I became unhappy. I lost contact with my friends as I had missed so much school. I thought I must have a serious illness as I felt so bad. My parents were really worried about me.

3. What did I do that made a difference?

   I started keeping a record of what I was doing each day and I was encouraged to gradually increase my activity. My exercise programme helped to build up my fitness and I felt less tired. I started eating regular meals again. I began to challenge my negative thoughts and I felt more positive. I made contact with my friends which really helped me to feel better.

4. How has my view of things changed?

   I no longer feel hopeless about the future in fact I am really pleased that I am going back to school.

5. How can I build on changes I have made?

   I need to continue pacing myself so that I don't overdo it and get tired. Making time to relax and go out with my friends is important.

6. What should I do if I relapse?

   I think it will be helpful to write down my activities and plan how to gradually build them up again. Stay positive and believe I can get over it.

The action plan for the future was fine-tuned in the review meeting. Further follow-up sessions were planned.

Conclusion

Chronic fatigue is an area where physiotherapists and occupational therapists are frequently asked to get involved. A graded activity approach can be helpful, but many patients are hampered by unhelpful thoughts and beliefs that make it hard to progress with their activity plan. A cognitive–behavioural approach, including graded activity, has a good evidence bases and is feasible for therapists with some basic training in CBT.

 ## Key Messages

- There is a wide variation in the prevalence of chronic fatigue syndrome reported in the literature.
- There are acceptable diagnostic criteria for CFS.
- There is good evidence for the use of CBT and graded exercise as key interventions in CFS.
- A shared approach by all members of the multidisciplinary team is essential.
- Family support for the treatment strategy is crucial for young people with CFS.

Sources of information accessible to patients

The internet

A search of one internet search engine using the keywords 'CFS', 'self-help' and 'patient advocacy' located more than 5,000 sites (Afari & Buchwald 2003).

Adults with CFS and parents of children with the condition often present clinicians with print-outs from the internet (Wright et al 1999). Of the thirteen websites Wright found, only six discussed rest and activity; only two of these recommended graded activity; two even recommended prolonged bed rest, which is known to be positively harmful (4–6 weeks' bed rest has been shown to result in 40% of loss of muscle strength (Bloomfield 1997)). Almost half of the websites made no mention of psychological support and one actively discouraged psychiatric input. Many gave details of diet, complementary therapies and pharmacological treatment, but there is limited research evidence on the benefits of these approaches (Wright et al 1999). In most studies immunological and antiviral substances have not been shown to be effective in the treatment of fatigue and other symptoms in CFS (Afari & Buchwald 2003).

Self-help groups

Another source of information about CFS is to be found in the literature provided by self-help groups, 'Action for ME' and 'the ME Association' (Macintyre 1998, Shepherd 1995, Shepherd & Chaudhuri 2001).

Disagreement between professionals and self-help organizations was highlighted in a CMO report into CFS (Sharpe 2002), although there is currently a considerable attempt to bring together different perspectives.

There is a suggestion in the literature that being a member of a support group can lead to poorer outcome (Sharpe et al 1992). However, there are clearly some patients who derive benefit from the support networks.

Sports instructors

The American College of Sports Science (Bailey 2003) suggests exercise activity should focus primarily on increasing the duration of moderate-intensity activities in preference to increasing exercise intensity. As stated above, bed rest and inactivity reduce muscle bulk and strength; inactivity will therefore only increase the impaired muscle function. Personal trainers may be very helpful, but their advice may need checking with current research.

Health professionals

Despite the evidence, many people are advised rest as a treatment by ill-informed health professionals (Chalder 1999).

Booklets

There are a number of self-help booklets available advocating a graded approach to exercise and other common sense advice. Examples of these are Chalder (1995) and Campling & Campling (2001).

Schools

In a small qualitative study (Everett & Fulton 2000) school teachers were shown to have some confusion over the available information on CFS, but to have some understanding of the physical and psychological components of the condition. The physiotherapist or occupational therapist may have a key role in liaising with schools, offering expert advice on exercise and activity, and in supporting students with CFS and their families as well as teachers.

References

Afari N, Buchwald D 2003 Chronic fatigue syndrome: a review. American Journal of Psychiatry 160:221–236

Bailey S 2003 Chronic fatigue syndrome. In: ACSM Exercise management for persons with chronic diseases and disabilities. Human Kinetics

Bloomfield S 1997 Changes in musculo-skeletal structure and function with prolonged bed rest. Medicine and Science in Sport and Exercise 29:197–206

Campling F, Campling J 2001 CFS – Your questions answered – a guide for newly diagnosed patients. Erskine Press

Carter B, Edwards J Kronenburger W et al 1995 Case control study of chronic fatigue in pediatric patients. Pediatrics 95(2): 179–186

Chalder T 1995 Coping with chronic fatigue. Sheldon Press, London

Chalder T 1999 Family orientated cognitive behaviour therapy for adolescents with CFS. In: Garralda E (ed) Chronic fatigue syndrome. Association for Child Psychology and Psychiatry Occasional Papers 16

Chalder T, Tong, Deary V 2002 Family cognitive behaviour therapy for chronic fatigue syndrome: an uncontrolled study. Archives of Diseases in Childhood 86:95–7

Chalder T, Goodman R, Wessely S et al 2003 Epidemiology of chronic fatigue syndrome and self reported myalgic encephalomyelitis in 5–15 year olds: cross sectional study. British Medical Journal 327:654

Cleare A J, Wessely S C 1996 Chronic fatigue syndrome: a stress disorder? British Journal of Hospital Medicine 55:571–574

Clements A, Sharpe M, Simkin S et al 1997 Chronic fatigue syndrome: a qualitative investigation of patients beliefs about the illness. Journal of Psychosomatic Research 42:615–624

David A, Wessely S, Pelosi A 1991 Chronic fatigue syndrome: signs of a new approach. British Journal of Hospital Medicine 45:158–163

Deale A, Chalder T, Marks I et al 1997 Cognitive behaviour therapy for chronic fatigue syndrome: a randomised controlled trial. American Journal of Psychiatry 154: 408–414

Deale A, Chalder T, Wessely S 1998 Illness beliefs and treatment outcome in chronic fatigue syndrome. Journal of Psychosomatic Research 45:77–83

Deale A, Husain K, Chalder T et al 2001 Long term outcome of CBT versus relaxation therapy for CFS: a 5 year follow-up study. American Journal of Psychiatry 158:2038–2042

Eminson M, Benjamin S, Shortall A et al 1996 Physical symptoms and illness attitudes in children and adolescents: an epidemiological study. Journal of Child Psychology and Psychiatry 37:519–528

Everett T, Fulton C 2000 An exploration of secondary school teachers' beliefs and attitudes about adolescent children with chronic fatigue syndrome. Unpublished MSc, Queen Margaret College, Edinburgh

Fukuda K, Straus E, Hickie I et al 1994 The chronic fatigue syndrome: a comprehensive approach to its definition and study. Annals of Internal Medicine 121:953–959

Fulcher K, White P 1997 Randomised controlled trial of graded exercise in patients with chronic fatigue syndrome. British Medical Journal 314:1647–1652

Fulcher K, White P 1998 Chronic fatigue syndrome a description of graded exercise treatment. Physiotherapy 84:223–226

Gallagher A M, Thompson J M, Hamilton W T et al 2004 Incidence of fatigue symptoms and diagnoses presenting in UK primary care from 1990 to 2001. Journal of the Royal Society of Medicine 97:571–576

Garralda E 1999 Chronic fatigue syndrome: helping children and adolescents. Association for Child Psychology and Psychiatry, Occasional Papers 1

Garralda E, Rangel L 2001 Childhood chronic fatigue syndrome. American Journal of Psychiatry 158:1161

Garralda E, Rangel L, Levin M et al 1999 Psychiatric adjustment in adolescents with a history of chronic fatigue syndrome. Journal of the American Academy of Child and Adolescent Psychiatry 38:1515–1521

Independent Working Group 2002 A report of the CFS/ME Working Group to the Chief Medical Officer. DOH, London

Jordan K, Landis D, Downey M et al 1998 Chronic fatigue syndrome in children and adolescents: a review. Journal of Adolescent Health 22:4–18

Joyce J, Hotopf M, Wessely S 1997 The prognosis of chronic fatigue and chronic fatigue syndrome: a systematic review. Quarterly Journal of Medicine 90:223–233

Lloyd A, Hickie I, Brockman A et al 1993 Immunologic and psychologic therapy for patients with chronic fatigue syndrome: a double-blind, placebo-controlled trial. American Journal of Medicine 94: 197–203

Macintyre A 1998 Chronic fatigue syndrome: a practical guide. Thorsons

Padesky C A 1994 Schema change processes in cognitive therapy. Clinical Psychology and Psychotherapy 1(5):267–278

Pemberton S, Hatcher S, Stanley P et al 1994 Chronic fatigue syndrome: a way forward. British Journal of Occupational Therapy 57:381–383

Powell P, Bentall R et al 2001 Randomised controlled trial of patient education to encourage graded exercise in chronic fatigue syndrome. British Medical Journal 322:387–390

Price J, Couper J 1999 Cognitive behaviour therapy for chronic fatigue syndrome in adults. The Cochrane Library Issue 2, Chichester

Price J, Couper J 2003 Cognitive behaviour therapy for chronic fatigue syndrome in adults (Cochrane Review). In the Cochrane Library, Issue 4, John Wiley, Chichester

Rangel L, Garralda M, Levin M et al 2000a The course of severe chronic fatigue syndrome in childhood. Journal of the Royal Society of Medicine 93:129–134

Rangel L, Garralda E, Levin M et al 2000b Personality in adolescents with chronic fatigue syndrome. European Child and Adolescent Psychiatry 9:39–45

Ray C, Jeffries S, Weir W 1995 Coping with chronic fatigue syndrome: illness responses and their relationship with fatigue, functional impairment and emotional status. Psychological Medicine 25:937–945

Sharpe M 2002 The report of the Chief Medical Officer's CSF/ME working group: what does it say and will it help? Clinical Medicine, Journal of the Royal College of Physicians 2(5):427–429

Sharpe M, Hawton K, Seagrott et al 1992 Follow-up of patients presenting with fatigue to an infectious diseases clinic. British Medical Journal 305:147–152

Sharpe M, Hawton K, Simkin S et al 1996 Cognitive therapy for chronic fatigue syndrome: a randomised controlled trial. British Medical Journal 312:22–36

Shepherd C 1995 Guidelines for the care of patients. 2nd edn. M E Association, Stanford-le-Hope, Essex

Shepherd C, Chaudhuri D 2001 ME/CFS/PVFS an exploration of the key clinical issues. The ME Association, Stanford-le-Hope, Essex

Theorell T, Blomvist V, Lindh, G et al 1999 Critical life events, infections and symptoms during the year preceding chronic fatigue syndrome (CFS): an examination of CFS patients and subjects with a non-specific life crisis. Psychosomatic Medicine 61: 304–310

Wessely S, Hotopf M, Sharpe M 1998 Chronic fatigue and its syndromes. Oxford University Press

White P, Naish V 2001 Graded exercise therapy for chronic fatigue syndrome: an audit. Physiotherapy 87(6):285–288

Whiting P, Bagnall A, Sowden A et al 2002 Interventions for the treatment and management of CFS: a systematic review. Journal of the American Medical Association 19, 286(11):1360–1368

Wilson A, Hickle I, Lloyd A et al 1994 Longitudinal study of the outcome of chronic fatigue syndrome. British Medical Journal 308:756–760

Wright B, Williams C, Partridge I 1999 Management advice for children with chronic fatigue syndrome: a systematic study of information from the internet. Irish Journal of Psychological Medicine 16:67–71

Concluding comments

Marie E Donaghy, Maggie Nicol and Kate Davidson

While pharmacological approaches and other forms of medical interventions are recognized as playing an important part in improving health outcomes, it is increasingly acknowledged that more holistic views of functioning and well-being require consideration of a whole systems approach. Therefore the role of psychosocial interventions needs to be strengthened within the health professional's therapeutic armamentarium in order to deliver more optimal health and social care. We believe that a thorough understanding of psychosocial approaches and their potential application, particularly cognitive–behavioural therapy (CBT) with its strong evidence base, needs to begin at pre-registration training for all health-care professionals and that psychosocial training should no longer be seen to be exclusive to the profession of psychology.

There is a variety of postgraduate opportunities to develop CBT expertise. These include CBT postgraduate degrees open to a range of health-care professionals and short courses which tend to be condition focused, for example CBT for chronic pain. Information on these programmes is available from a variety of sources such as local health board information leaflets and websites, professional body websites and from the British Association of Behavioural and Cognitive Psychotherapy (BABCP). These programmes allow people to get a basic training, but further competence in delivering CBT is required through supervision with an experienced cognitive–behavioural therapist. The move towards interdisciplinary working should open the doors to cross-professional supervision within teams where appropriate. If we are seriously going to improve health- and social-care outcomes we need to embrace a multi-professional learning environment and increase our willingness to share our expertise and learn together.

The chapters within this book illustrate how CBT can add value to current treatments in regard to optimizing health-care outcomes. There is a need for occupational therapists and physiotherapists and other health-care professions to consider the application of CBT within their traditional professional models and to evaluate the efficacy using appropriate research methodologies in order to create and strengthen the evidence base.

The roots of CBT lie in mental disorders, such as anxiety and depression, recognizing that mood is regulated through cognition and behaviour and the interaction between these systems, with the greatest body of treatment efficacy relating to this area. In recent years the use of CBT has been extended to other clinical areas where there is a comorbid mood disorder associated with other clinical conditions such as pain, fibromyalgia and chronic fatigue, with a growing body of evidence for its treatment efficacy.

The authors propose that there are opportunities for occupational therapists and physiotherapists to extend cognitive–behavioural approaches into areas where there is no apparent mood disorder but where alteration to particular psychological constructs, such as how one views oneself, how one views the world, and how one views the future, is triggered by illness, accident, disease or social circumstances. The effects of these alterations can have a wide impact, for example on self-esteem, body image, family and social relationships. Occupational therapists and physiotherapists, especially those working more within the physical domains of practice, may be very well placed to adapt the cognitive–behavioural model to these types of disorders, offering a more complete patient/client-focused health-care service.

Taking this forward may present challenges for occupational therapists and physiotherapists to consider in more specific detail psychological perspectives which may limit or inhibit recovery. We would recommend that one way to take this forward is to consider the techniques, approaches and applications presented in the different chapters in Part Two of this book, for example cognitive restructuring, managing worry, monitoring behaviour through experiments and homework, and keeping a diary, and to consider their application in different areas of practice.

The authors are not advocating that occupational therapists and physiotherapists lose their uni-professional identity and become cognitive–behavioural therapists; rather that cognitive–behavioural approaches would add a useful extra dimension to their practice. We would recommend that occupational therapists and physiotherapists consider developing their knowledge, competencies and skills in CBT as part of their continuing professional development.

Appendix
Guided discovery and the Socratic approach

The key elements to guided discovery are forming a collaborative basis to work, guiding the patient to find the answer, seeing the patient as the expert and helping him/her to learn skills strategies so that he/she can rely on himself/herself rather than the therapist.

A Socratic questioning style is helpful in promoting guided discovery. The essence of this approach is that the therapist encourages curiosity about how things are; in a process that involves questioning, listening and summarizing, the therapist draws attention to new information which can help the patient evaluate previous ways of thinking or develop new ways of thinking.

Useful questions in the Socratic approach

* What went through your head?
* What do you think about that?
* What does that mean to you?
* What is the evidence for that?
* How else can you think about it?
* What else do you think?
* How do you explain that?
* What are the disadvantages/advantages of your choice?
* What is your understanding of that?
* If that were true, what would that mean to you?
* If someone else said that to you, how would you reply?

Index

169

175